A SOCIAL HISTORY OF MEDICINE

A *Social History of Medicine* traces the development of medical practice over a period of enormous change, from the Industrial Revolution right through to the twentieth century. Drawing on a wide range of source material, it charts the changing relationship between patients and practitioners over this period, exploring the impact made by institutional care, government intervention and scientific discovery.

The study illuminates the extent to which medical assistance was genuinely available for all patients during the period by drawing on local sources and focusing on the provinces. The author introduces a number of hitherto unknown contemporary medical practitioners, and gives fascinating details of their work.

The text offers an extensive thematic survey, including coverage of:

- institutions such as hospitals, dispensaries, asylums and prisons
- midwifery and nursing
- infections, and the impact of science on disease control
- contraception, war and the establishment of the NHS.

A *Social History of Medicine* provides an engaging introduction to the subject which will appeal to students and teachers alike.

Joan Lane is a Senior Teaching Fellow in History at the University of Warwick. She is also the author of *Apprenticeship in England, 1600-1914* (UCL Press, 1996) and *The Making of the English Patient* (2000).

A SOCIAL HISTORY OF MEDICINE

Health, healing and disease in England, 1750–1950

Joan Lane

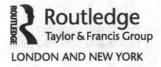

Routledge
Taylor & Francis Group

LONDON AND NEW YORK

First published 2001
by Routlege
4 Park Square, Milton Park, Abingdon, Oxon OX14 4RN
605 Third Avenue, New York, NY 10017

Routledge is an imprint of the Taylor & Francis Group,
an informa business

Typeset in Goudy by Saxon Graphics Ltd, Derby

British Library Cataloguing in Publication Data
A catalogue record for this book is available from the British Library

Library of Congress Cataloging in Publication Data

Lane, Joan
    A social history of medicine in England, 1750-1950 / Joan Lane.
        p. cm.
    Includes bibliographical references and index.
        1. Medicine–England–History. 2. Medical care–Social
aspects–England–History. 3.
    Health–Social aspects–England–History. 4. Social
medicine–England–History. I.
    Title.

R487 .L36 2001
610′.942–dc21
00-062758

ISBN 13: 978-0-415-20038-7 (pbk)
ISBN 13: 978-0-415-20038-7 (hbk)

CONTENTS

ILLUSTRATIONS

TABLES

PREFACE

The social history of medicine in England is, by any standards, the history of every inhabitant. As we all experience birth, illness, ageing and death, we all become patients at one time or another, in the care of various branches of medicine, as did most of our ancestors. The changes that socialised medicine have brought in the last half century are perhaps the most sweeping in modern British history, although in the two centuries from 1750 to 1950 medical practice itself changed out of all recognition. At a time of unequalled population growth, industrialisation and economic advance, the consumer society demanded more from medicine and practitioners than merely to ease the pathway to death. Medicine responded with new drugs and techniques alongside its own growth in numbers and prosperity, leading to an enhanced status as a profession that would have been inconceivable in early Georgian England.

This book has been written to try to bring together the significant themes and developments in medicine as part of social history, as part of all our lives, past and present. It has grown from the course I teach in the History Department at the University of Warwick and I am grateful to students on the course during two decades for their involvement and to colleagues for helpful discussions over the years. Readers may find an emphasis on the provinces, and especially on the Midlands and midland archives, but this is 'the land where I belong' and where much of my research has been carried out. We no longer need convincing that all history is local history. The Midlands is also the birthplace of the Industrial Revolution and where a number of significant developments and personalities influenced medical practice: innovations such as Lilley Smith's dispensaries or medical giants such as William Withering and Erasmus Darwin.

At the end of each chapter I have included transcripts of original material to show the richness and variety of medical sources, but also to illustrate how archives are the true basis of research, even though much has been lost in two centuries. I have also added a section on further reading, rather than individually footnoting every source. The index of medical names gives each practitioner's dates, rather than interrupting the main text to include this information, and place names in the index are given in their historic county, before the 'reorganisation' of 1974.

I have become indebted to many record offices and their archivists during my research, especially those in the Midlands, to the RAF Museum at Hendon and to the Wellcome Institute in London for their never-failing helpfulness to my many enquiries. Jonathan Reinarz has kindly examined material there for me and

Len Smith has provided valuable advice on county lunatic asylums. The Wellcome Trust has also supported my research into friendly societies and into Poor Law medicine over the years. I am grateful to Ann Bennett for skilfully producing photographs. I would also like to thank the private owners of manuscripts, portraits and photographs who have so willingly allowed me to use their material.

Note

Pre-decimal currency

1s (shilling) = 5p
1d (penny) is a twelfth part of a shilling
A guinea (£1 1s) = £1.05p

ACKNOWLEDGEMENT

'Diary of an NHS baby', by George Pendle, first appeared in *The Times* 23 June 1998 and is reproduced with the permission of News International © George Pendle/Times Newspapers Ltd, 23 June 1998.

INTRODUCTION

MEDICINE BEFORE THE INDUSTRIAL REVOLUTION

Edward Rawlins, aged about two years, had a hard Tumor
of one of his Stones to the bigness of a Hen's Egg, which
was cured as followeth: ℞ Linseeds, powder them, and
with Linseed Oil make a Pultess, which was applied hot.
After there was a little Bag made of Cloth to keep it up in,
with which he was cured.

John Hall, *Select Observations on English Bodies*, 1679 edn, p. 52

The way in which John Hall, a physician and son-in-law of William Shakespeare, treated a local gentleman's son for a testicular swelling in many ways typifies qualified medical practice before the mid-eighteenth century. Medicine was really available only to the prosperous, provided by a small band of practitioners and based on a mixture of Galenical and chemical remedies. Diagnosis was imperfect and there was no understanding of how infections were transmitted, while bleeding and purging were the standard techniques even the weakest patients endured. Although there was general acceptance that the patient's mind might affect the state of physical health, there was no grasp of psychological illness beyond categorising sufferers as 'manic' and 'melancholic'. Qualified medical practitioners formed a pyramid of three distinct groups – physicians, surgeons and apothecaries. At the top, physicians were university-educated men, usually holding the degree of MD, but actually having studied only non-medical subjects at university, such as philosophy; the rarest of all the practitioners, they advised patients, suggested remedies and charged high fees. Surgeons, separated from the barbers in 1540, were trained by traditional apprenticeship and carried out manual tasks, such as amputations or lancing boils. Apothecaries, also apprenticed, dispensed and sold medicines, often in their shops; the most numerous of the groups, they were allowed to charge only for the pills or powders they dispensed, not for the advice they usually provided.

Although all practitioners were relatively scarce in England in proportion to the population as a whole, expectation of life before the early eighteenth century was so low (thirty-seven for men, often less for women) that professional skills

1

were summoned only in the great crises of life and death. Most illnesses were treated in the home and children were rarely attended by a medical practitioner. Childbirth was entirely the midwife's responsibility, with help from the patient's female relatives, even in the highest ranks of society. Accidents, such as fractures, however, did require a surgeon's attention and John Hall's casebook shows the range of serious ailments a high-status physician might treat, including syphilis, tuberculosis, puerperal fever and cirrhosis of the liver, as well as lesser afflictions (catarrh, constipation and migraine), travelling across a large area of the Midlands to do so. When epidemics struck, formal medicine had no effective response and in outbreaks of sweating sickness, typhus ('spotted fever', 'gaol fever'), plague or smallpox, patients frequently resorted to unqualified empirics or quacks. Not surprisingly, traditional potions were tried, many relying on sympathetic magic for effect (frogspawn for leucorrhoea, red blankets for smallpox). When a new infection struck, there was no natural immunity and all levels of society were afflicted, so that Henry VII's son, Prince Arthur, died of sweating sickness in 1502, James I's son of typhus in 1612 and Queen Mary of smallpox in 1694.

The practice of medicine in early modern England was dominated by the humoral theory, originating in ancient Greece. There were thought to be four cardinal humours – blood, phlegm, choler (yellow bile) and melancholy (black bile). Galen of Pergamon associated these with the elements of air (blood was warm and moist), water (phlegm was cold and moist), fire (yellow bile was warm and dry) and earth (black bile was cold and dry). In each individual and each part of the body there was a natural combination of these humours and when one humour was dominant in a patient, upsetting the desired balance, illness would follow. Thus, when blood (air) predominated, the patient had a sanguine disposition, a ruddy complexion and an optimistic outlook, while when black bile (earth) was dominant, the individual would have a dark complexion, thin physique and meditative outlook, given to melancholy. The practitioner's task was to restore the humoral balance by using medicines with qualities opposite those of the excessive humour – a hot, dry drug for a phlegmatic patient, for example. The range of diseases that could afflict a patient was vividly described by Thersites in *Troilus and Cressida* (V, i):

> Now, the rotten diseases of the south, the guts-griping ruptures, catarrhs, loads o' gravel in the back, lethargies, cold palsies, raw eyes, dirt-rotten livers, wheezing lungs, bladders full of imposthume, sciaticas, limekilns i' the palm, incurable bone ache ...

Patients could be purged, bled and made to vomit or sweat. Medicines could be given as pills, powders, syrups, ointments and plasters. Most preparations were polypharmaceutical, made with a very large number of ingredients from which the body would select what the disease required, again based on Galen's theories, and on the *Pharmacopoeia Londonensis*, prepared by the London College of

Physicians, which first appeared in 1618 by order of James I. In pre-industrial England, as in later years, personal accidents were always a threat, but the medieval and early modern periods seem dominated by great epidemics, bubonic plague, the 'sweating sickness', leprosy, typhus and smallpox, the last two of which were to flourish for centuries, to be joined in the nineteenth century by cholera and typhoid. Apart from public health measures, medicine was to reduce only one of these scourges, smallpox, before the present century, although others became less virulent (plague) or disappeared (sweating sickness and leprosy).

It is widely accepted that, before the Dissolution of the Monasteries by Henry VIII in 1537, the sparse medical services that did exist in England were provided by members of the religious orders. The hospital of St Peter and St Leonard in York, founded in 936, as a general establishment for the relief of the poor, including the sick, is considered to be the earliest. However, this makes no recognition of the non-religious, especially surgeons, who practised independently. The suppression of the parochial guilds ten years later also greatly reduced medical and welfare provisions for the population as a whole, for these fraternities ran hospitals, schools and almshouses for their members; Birmingham's Holy Cross guild provided the services of a midwife, for example. However, from the twelfth century, well before the Dissolution, there had existed a network of specialist hospitals for sufferers from one particular disease, leprosy, where patients were attended but kept away from the rest of society, well beyond the outskirts of a town or city; perhaps the first example of socially managing a disease. The total number of these lazar houses has been given as over four hundred; four have been identified in Derbyshire, for example, but after 1350 leprosy declined and by the mid-fifteenth century few were functioning. The buildings were then used for the general relief of poverty and increasingly to isolate pauper syphilis sufferers, as the disease became more common. The reasons for the decline of leprosy, a dreaded infection, are obscure; the isolation policy must have played an important part, the disease may have lost its virulence and mis-diagnosis (mistaking leprosy for other skin complaints, for example) must have occurred. Amazingly, some lazar houses can still be seen, surviving as almshouses (St Mary Magdalene, Ripon, founded in 1139 for eighteen patients), as modern places of worship (Rochester Hospital at Chatham, St John's at Northampton, Domus Dei at Portsmouth) and occasionally as an infirmary (Christ's Hospital, near Durham, founded in 1181 for sixty-five inmates). Others have become sad ruins (the master's house of St Michael's, Warwick or St Margaret's, Taunton) and the leper's squint has survived in very few parish churches. Perhaps the most permanent commemoration of a leper house can be seen in the Leicestershire place-name of Burton Lazars, where the hospital, founded by the Knights of the Order of St Lazarus of Jerusalem between 1138 and 1162, had waterways and a moat for patients' hydrotherapy.

However, it is clear that medical attention from physicians and surgeons continued to suffering individuals between the Dissolution and the Industrial Revolution. As early as 1570–90 there were seventy-three practitioners to attend the 17,000 population of Norwich, while twenty-four practised in Ipswich and fifteen in King's Lynn in the second half of the sixteenth century. A modern survey from 1603 to 1643 has shown 814 physicians scattered across the countryside, with 15 in Northamptonshire, 58 in Devon and 27 in Yorkshire, for example. Even after the disruptions of the Civil War, bishops continued to license medical practitioners. Thus in the period 1661–1712 in Warwickshire, for instance, there were thirty-six licences granted (twenty-nine to surgeons, seven to physicians) and forty-seven in Worcestershire (forty surgeons, seven physicians). The growth of institutional care for poorer patients, however, was very slow indeed, even in London, and non-existent in the provinces. Infectious diseases undoubtedly terrified society and although temporary pesthouses were established in England for plague and smallpox victims, it was not until after the Restoration that purpose-built hospitals were erected; St Mary's of Bethlehem (Bedlam) in 1675–6 and St Thomas's (rebuilt in 1693–1709), both in London.

Although most English provincial hospitals were founded in the 1740s and 50s, they were following a pattern already existing in London, where, apart from St Thomas's and St Bartholomew's Hospitals (both refounded after the Dissolution), five new infirmaries were built in the period 1720–45, Westminster (1720), Guy's (1724), St George's (1733), the London (1740) and the Middlesex (1745). In the provinces the development was slower but steady, so that by 1800 only seventeen of the thirty-nine English counties did not have an infirmary, including three (Essex, Middlesex and Surrey) that were close to the London institutions and in twenty-two counties there were in fact twenty-nine hospitals (see Chapter 5).

Asylums for the insane followed a similar pattern. In the period before the mid-fifteenth century, institutions were not provided for them and even Bedlam originally admitted general patients as well as lunatics. However, by the early seventeenth century there were small private madhouses where the physically violent could be lodged and supervised, although a public institution was not to be established until the early eighteenth century when a clergy widow, Mary Chapman, founded the first 'public Bethel' in the provinces at Norwich in 1713 (see Chapter 6).

It might be thought that, before the Industrial Revolution, occupational diseases would be few and rare, with handicrafts, domestic workshops and agricultural labour providing safer, less polluted livelihoods than factories, machinery and dangerous new raw materials. However, in the first medical textbook to deal with occupational health, A Treatise on the Diseases of Tradesmen (1706), Bernard Ramazzini covered such traditional workmen as the baker, carpenter, saddler and blacksmith among the forty-three categories of those he considered at risk from their occupations. Translated from Latin into English in 1726 by Dr Robert James, it went into several editions and remained a standard text for decades. At the centre of eighteenth-century industrialisation, midland medical practitioners were early writers on occupational diseases. Thus Thomas Tomlinson (The

Medical Miscellany, 1769) and William Richardson (*Chemical Principles of the Metallic Arts*, 1790), both Birmingham surgeons, wrote vividly of the area's workers and their health. Well into the next century, John Darwall, also of Birmingham, chose *Diseases of Artisans* as the title of his Edinburgh MD thesis in 1821.

Ramazzini condemned sedentary work, repetitive strain injuries (weavers suffered from 'pain in the loins') and the raw materials used (bakers' and millers' eyes were bleary from flour particles), while even skilled men such as watchmakers endured gradual loss of sight from the closeness of their tasks. In addition, before the Industrial Revolution brought steam power, much work relied entirely on human strength, as in building, metal work and mining, and many men suffered, especially from hernias, and even died from their exertions. Heavy weights, sharp tools, falls and accidents were common causes of injury in the majority of occupations, compounded in some cases by alcohol.

It is not surprising that a wide range of occupations was well-known, even notorious, for having hard-drinking workers. Men who worked in very hot conditions and sweated profusely needed liquid to survive. The brazier, glassblower, plumber and tallow chandler were all known as heavy drinkers, as was the plasterer, whose work involved mixing large quantities of slaked lime and sand. Again, in the strength trades, such as those of the stonemason, blacksmith or nailer, alcohol was thought to replace the worker's vigour, lost through his physical effort and sweat. Even in occupations that were not hot or dusty, beer was an accepted part of the workshop culture, essential in an apprentice's initiation and when the term was completed. It is clear that, before the Industrial Revolution and the coming of factories, beer was regularly drunk by all levels of tradesmen at the workplace and, indeed, alternatives would have been hard to find in town or country. Water was generally not safe to drink and milk was exclusively for infants and invalids. Tea and coffee, at this early period, of course, were expensive, fashionable beverages not available to workers. In some rural areas there were local alternatives to ale; cider was consumed in the West Country and Herefordshire, perry in Worcestershire.

With the coming of industrialisation and increased productivity to meet growing consumerism, workers used many new processes and raw materials, some of them highly dangerous. Although glaziers and painters had long been at risk of nerve damage (palsy) from using lead, after the mid-eighteenth century the demands for their services grew with the expansion in building, as new Georgian houses required more piping and plumbing, sinks and windows than architecture of an earlier period. Later the popularity of beaver hats, which needed treating with mercury and sulphur, 'heated rather higher than unpractised hands could bear', was blamed for the trade's brain-damaged workers and the source of the phrase 'mad as a hatter'. Sometimes, a craftsman might be aware of the risks in his trade and, as early as 1683, Nicholas Paris worried at the dangers of using too much aqua fortis (nitric acid) as he regilded the great tomb of Richard Beauchamp in Warwick:

I could have hartily wished that I had gave a hondred pound so that I
had not ever medled with it for it hath done me more harme that ever
I shall get by it, for it hath cost me allmost my life twise a bout the doing
of it as the Docters will aferme.

In spite of his worries, Paris did not die until 1716, aged about seventy.

Although deafness increased with the coming of machinery in factories, even
such a traditional worker as the miller suffered loss of hearing from the noise of
grinding corn, while 'weavers' deafness' was common into the twentieth century.
A polluted environment was a constant hazard and early in the eighteenth
century Ramazzini had noted the 'killing smell' endured by the tallow chandler,
oilman and tanner, describing their complexion as 'death-like' and their appearance as splenetic and puffed-up. Later damage to the lungs was common in
textile factories, where 'flew' (cotton down) filled the air and windows, required
under the 1802 Factory Act, were kept firmly closed. Needle making and the
cutlery trades produced fine metal and stone particles, causing fatal lung damage,
as did all forms of mining. Darwall observed that the 'air of the factories is completely loaded with dust, and the workmen cannot avoid inhaling it'. Although
reformers to stop children from climbing chimneys were active in eighteenth-
century England, climbing boys were a minority of young workers. However, as
cases of death from suffocation and burning were given wide publicity, reforms
were eventually achieved, although relatively little public attention was given to
the damning medical evidence presented to a Parliamentary Select Committee
in 1816 that climbing boys suffered from scrotal and lip cancer as a result of constant contact with soot. Very young and thus small children were, of course,
required for sweeping chimneys, as they were in factories where they worked as
'pieceners', joining broken threads together and able to crawl under the looms to
do so.

Hippocrates had recognised that there were 'very many Arts and Callings
which are useful and pleasant to those who stand in need of their Assistance, but
occasion a great deal of Trouble and Labour to those who practise them'. He had
not, moreover, considered the extremely long working day of most occupations;
twelve hours were always worked, fourteen hours were common. A six-day week
was universal and, when extra productivity was required to meet a large order,
even longer hours would be necessary. In addition, apprenticeship meant that
men and women would stay for life in the occupation to which they had been
indentured, no matter how unhealthy. Thus long hours exacerbated the health
risks of their trade for all workers, especially the young, and physical deformity
was inevitable; in the Black Country nailing made the workman's one shoulder
higher than the other and the area was nick-named 'Humpshire' because of it.

Although Ramazzini recommended various foods to soothe and reduce the
irritant effects of some occupations, there was no medical discussion of protec-
tive clothing until William Richardson, a Birmingham surgeon, wrote of his own
experiences in 1790 when treating sick workers in the local industries. He sug-

gested that they should 'put on something like a waggoner's frock at work, laying [it] aside when they have done'. He also recommended washing after finishing work and before eating, but writers noted that workers would usually not do so and facilities were generally lacking. The most significant medical text on occupational health was Charles Turner Thackrah's *The Effects of the Principal Arts, Trades and Professions ... on Health and Longevity*, of which an expanded second edition appeared in 1831, noted in the local press and favourably reviewed in medical journals. A chemist's son from Leeds, Thackrah had trained at Guy's Hospital, a fellow student of John Keats, and his return to practise in Leeds coincided with the founding of the town's medical school. Although other treatises had been written at this period about single occupational diseases (John Darwall on grinders' asthma in the Black Country and Charles Hastings on bronchitis in Worcester china workers), Thackrah's covered a very wide range of diseases and some 177 trades. He noted dangerous substances (dust, chemicals) and working conditions (odours, posture, temperatures), as well as the risks to females of wearing stays and the generally poor housing conditions and environment which most workers endured. He was also aware of the mental stress that professional men experienced, an aspect of their lives that can be seen in many contemporary diaries. Having served as Leeds town surgeon, Thackrah died from pulmonary tuberculosis in 1833 aged only thirty-eight.

The risks for those who worked with animals were virtually ignored by the population at large, although a number of deaths brought before coroners were the result of animal accidents (6.7 per cent in Wiltshire in 1752–96, for example). There were obvious dangers from handling animals; horses could bolt or throw their riders, cattle could trample or gore their stockmen, all creatures could bite and every level of society was in closer contact with animals in the eighteenth and nineteenth centuries than is usually appreciated. Farriers, blacksmiths and veterinary surgeons were all at risk from zoonotic infections, of which glanders was the most feared. Charles Vial de St Bel, founder of the London Veterinary College, died from the disease in 1793, but less fatal hazards such as ringworm remained until well into the twentieth century for those who worked with animals. Tradesmen who prepared animal skins to be used for leather products, such as the woolcomber or tanner, were at risk from anthrax, usually fatal, and nick-named 'woolsorter's disease'.

The general public, however, in contact with animals, were also susceptible to such zoonotic infections as rabies, tetanus (lockjaw) and leptospirosis (Weil's disease), all of which resulted in extremely unpleasant deaths. Of these, there were innumerable but ineffectual cures for hydrophobia (rabies) and livelihoods to be made from selling such remedies. Perhaps the best-known rabies treatment was Colne Medicine, made and sold by a Lancashire landowner, Robert Parker, and widely praised. Initially it sold at the high price of 2s. 6d. a bottle, later reduced to a shilling. The range of customers for this preparation, both in geographical area (from Durham to Derbyshire) and social class, was remarkable, with some 1,500 doses sold in a decade, evenly divided between humans and animals.

What made sufferers choose empirical remedies, rather than follow the qualified practitioner's advice, could have been desperation in seeking a cure, the difference in cost and even the difficulty of securing the services of a surgeon-apothecary or physician in the early part of the eighteenth century. However, as the numbers of qualified practitioners had grown substantially by about 1760, adequately covering the country, the decision to seek quack advice must have been taken for other reasons, including a rising standard of living in a consumerist society. Undoubtedly, the empirics advertised their services and wares aggressively. Roy Porter has described their activities at this period as 'medical entrepreneurship' and it is clear that they were providing a service in response to popular demand. Their press advertisements list the range of distressing ailments, many chronic, for which cures were needed and for which the medical profession had few treatments. In regional newspapers they printed recommendations from named patients and there is substantial evidence from contemporary letters and diaries that educated, prosperous patients mixed quack with orthodox remedies in 'a lively medical pluralism'.

The empirics travelled the provinces to promote their cures, and the wide range of their services in an area can be judged from one typical local newspaper of the period. In *Jopson's Coventry Mercury* during the middle decades of the eighteenth century some of the empirics who advertised included Dr Uytrecht and Carl Goergsleiner (oculists), Dr Nash of Bromsgrove (uroscopist), Dr Timon ('famous London operator for the ears'), Mr R. B. Shapee ('cures ruptures and fallen womb') and Signior Grimaldi (dentist). Sometimes their services became unnecessary as technology advanced; thus, hernia operations had long been the quacks' province, with an almost inevitable risk of castration, but improved trusses by the early eighteenth century were an effective non-surgical solution. Many of these charlatans had or acquired foreign names and invariably advertised the local inn at which they could be consulted. In addition, many remedies were widely available and sold in various shops, especially a bookseller's, milliner's, draper's or newspaper office, rather than in an apothecary's, again extending the range of non-professional medical treatments that could be purchased, often for pennies. There is also substantial evidence in the accounts of the Overseers of the Poor at this period that such remedies were bought for sick paupers, alongside the formal attention provided by the parish surgeon, as well as the services of the bonesetter, uroscopist and oculist. Typical of such preparations and how they were advertised, an increasingly important aspect of quackery, was Godfrey's Cordial, which sold for 6d in 1748, and was promoted as:

> so universally approved for all Manner of Pains in the Bowels, Fluxes, Fevers, Small Pox, Measles, Rheumatism, Coughs, Colds and Restlessness in Men, Women and Children, and particularly for Several Ailments incident to Child-Bearing Women, and Relief of Young Children in Breeding their Teeth.

8

Dr Benjamin Godfrey described himself as having an MD and a warehouse in London. His product was later said to contain sassafras, syrup and opium.

Some of these alternative practitioners were very prosperous indeed, especially in London, and attracted considerable envy from the qualified. Mrs Sally Mapp, the Epsom bonesetter, Chevalier John Taylor, the oculist, and Joshua Ward, a former drysalter, all vividly depicted by Hogarth in his *Company of Undertakers* (1737), became extremely wealthy as a result of their skills. Preparations for the eyes and ears were favourite products for quacks, although the richest pickings and the greatest demand for cures were in the treatment of sexual problems, especially male impotence and unwanted pregnancies, while cures for venereal infections were numerous and profitable throughout the eighteenth and nineteenth centuries. By 1783, the government were devising a tax on 'quacks and vendors of nostrums' and a tax on patent medicines that was capable of yielding about £15,000 a year.

The line between charlatan and orthodox was not always clear, for a number of qualified practitioners, such as John Pechey or John Taylor, also made lucrative livings as quacks, while William Read was knighted by Queen Anne. In addition, some distinguished qualified men, such as Robert James, Hans Sloane, Richard Mead and Edward Jenner, also promoted remedies bearing their names, usually in the more expensive range of preparations. However, most qualified practitioners considered that quacks threatened their professional livelihoods and sought to discredit them whenever possible, although often employing their techniques of advertising and even the same basic ingredients.

The problems of fertility dominated the eighteenth-century medical fringe market. Failure to conceive was clearly seen as a woman's fault, although male impotence was an acknowledged difficulty for which many cures were sold. Some advertisements claimed that the products, while not directly promoted as abortifacients, would remove 'female obstructions' and renew menstruation, while others were said to aid conception. The most notorious character in the medical sex market was James Graham, a showman who claimed to be qualified, the 'Master Quack' whose Celestial Bed and Temple of Hymen were intended to promote conception, where 'children of the most perfect beauty could be begotten'. A successful speaker, enthusiast for electricity and self-publicist, he used dramatic visual effects to attract clients, charging 50 guineas a night in the Celestial Bed to conquer sexual debility.

Early eighteenth-century England saw medicine struggle to be more orthodox and indeed a recognisable medical profession had emerged by the early 1800s. The numbers of practitioners had grown, as had the population they attended, but consumerist Georgian society and its rising expectations increasingly sought professional attention for various medical conditions that had formerly been endured or treated at home. Although England was undeniably a more hazardous place to live and work with the coming of industrialisation, society devised more institutional provisions for workers, as hospitals, dispensaries and friendly societies multiplied throughout the eighteenth century. Also, the great epidemics of earlier periods, such as plague and sweating sickness, had disappeared, while the scourge of smallpox was to be lessened by the use of inoculation. In addition, a higher standard of living and fewer great harvest failures, along with better transport and agrarian improvements, meant that society at large was, however slowly, moving towards lower death rates and a healthier population, while medical skills and techniques continued to improve.

Occupational risks at work

A farm servant at Longworth, Herefordshire, fell from a hayrick onto the staff of a dray that he was about to load, the staff, which was sharp, went through his belly and back. He cleared himself from it, and carried his Intrails in his Hands 20 Yards for Assistance, but died the next Morning.

Berrow's Worcester Journal, 2 April 1747

Last Wednesday morning the following melancholy Accident happened at Ormesby, a Village about five Miles from Yarmouth. As the Son of Mr Clowes, a Wheelwright, a Lad about 14 Years old, was in a Malt Mill belonging to his Uncle, the Mill suddenly caught hold of him under his Chin, and threw him upon the Cogs, which in a few Minutes (there being no body at Hand) tore him to Pieces in a most miserable Manner, leaving him hardly a Bone whole about him. He expired immediately.

Aris's Birmingham Gazette, 12 June 1758

Dangers for gilders at work, 1790

Gilders should be particularly cautious to turn their heads aside as much as can be during their work; for by properly attending to this, they would escape most of the fumes. They should moreover always contrive, as much as possible, by opening the windows, or door of the place where they are at work, to have a current of air from behind them towards the chimney. Where this could be managed, especially if a brisk fire were at the same time kept up, the mercurial fumes, instead of being diffused in the atmosphere around them, would be immediately carried away in a body up the chimney.

With regard to the diet of such people, it should be nourishing, but quite temperate. Whenever they feel themselves much disordered, they should take a vomit; and they should always be careful to keep their bodies [bowels] moderately open.

William Richardson,
The Chemical Principles of the Metallic Arts, 1790, p. 198

1

MEDICAL PRACTITIONERS IN EIGHTEENTH- AND NINETEENTH-CENTURY ENGLAND

I studied hard; learned the Linnean names and doses of drugs; attended seven surgical operations; worked from nine to nine daily, Sundays included; made mercury ointment in the old style by turning a pestle in a mortar for three days in succession, to amalgamate the quicksilver with the pig's grease; made up what the doctor called his 'Cathartic acid bitter mixture', as a sort of fill-up for every purgative bottle, and almost every disease that 'flesh is heir to'; made up boluses ... drew a tooth for sixpence ... did many things during that six months which gave me a distaste for the practice of medicine ...

J. Clegg (ed.), *Autobiography of a Lancashire Lawyer* [John Taylor], 1883

The provision of medical attention since the early modern period in England had always been a business, with fees paid for services rendered. However, in the consumerist eighteenth century, medicine expanded fastest of all the superior occupations to become, by the Victorian period, a recognised and respected profession, with registration, professional journals and a career structure in both private practice and institutional appointments. In the early years of the eighteenth century all medical practitioners, physicians, surgeons and apothecaries, were few in proportion to the population as a whole, their unscientific treatments were invariably unsuccessful and, significantly, patients were not disposed to seek and pay for advice except in desperate circumstances. By the 1750s, however, patients increasingly came to spend money on more scientific successful medical attention as part of a higher standard of living, greater disposable income and increased life expectancy. Medicine became, with larger apprenticeship premiums, better incomes and higher social status for practitioners, an occupation which gentry or ambitious parents could choose as a career for their sons. It was an exclusively male occupation until the present century. A number of physicians had fathers who were clergy (William Small, Clifton Wintringham) and landowners (Richard Wilkes, John Johnstone). The profession's status was undeniably improved when the surgeons separated from the more menial barbers in 1745. The period produced some very grand, wealthy and famous practitioners to inspire the young apprentice or pupil as role models.

There was a significant dividing-line in Georgian England between physicians, as university-trained men, and those who had been apprenticed, the surgeons and the apothecaries. The physicians attended the universities of Oxford, Cambridge, Glasgow, Edinburgh, St Andrews or Aberdeen to gain the qualification of MD and the privileged title of 'Doctor'; Edinburgh was particularly popular in the eighteenth century, especially when continental travel became more difficult. All non-Anglicans, whose religious beliefs barred them from British universities, might train on the continent, chiefly at Leiden, Rheims or Padua, and then practise as physicians at home, although a foreign training was clearly less favoured by the 1760s. Physicians remained at the apex of the medical pyramid, few in number, practising only in the largest towns and cities, charging high fees and accepted as gentlemen. They saw patients, gave advice and recommended treatments, but generally never performed manual tasks or dispensed medications. Surgeons and apothecaries, although originally separate occupations, increasingly joined their skills into the title of surgeon-apothecary, the equivalent of the modern general practitioner. However, specialists in these distinct branches of medicine continued to practise, especially in hospitals, while apothecaries also ran retail businesses. Apprenticeship was the means by which both became qualified through a system that had existed in England since the Norman Conquest; it was illegal to practise most occupations if unapprenticed. As an apprentice, a youth was bound for a term, usually for seven years at the age of fourteen, by his parents or guardians to a qualified master, to whom they paid a lump sum, the premium, to cover the boy's tuition, board and lodging while he was indentured. The medical apprentice clearly had to be literate and numerate, with a basic grasp of Latin. Although many apprenticeships were arranged through personal connections and by word of mouth, by the 1750s, as medicine expanded and attracted new recruits, advertising for apprentices in the local press was common, the master's name not usually disclosed. The youth lived in the master's house as part of the family and was not paid; the indenture demanded certain standards of behaviour from the apprentice and placed strict limits on his personal behaviour while he was indentured. Residence with the master was an important part of medical training, especially for hospital pupils, so that John Keats lodged with Astley Cooper, who had earlier boarded with Henry Cline.

The premium was the critical factor in deciding what career a boy might pursue, essentially what his parents could afford. Premiums were always higher in London, provincial cities and fashionable watering places, where masters could charge patients larger fees. Also, eminent men could command far bigger premiums, so that, for example, Caesar Hawkins, surgeon at St George's Hospital, took £200 with a Lancashire gentleman's son in 1736, while William Cheselden, the famous lithotomist, accepted £150, £210 and £350 with three apprentices in the years 1712–30, sums only just below those paid to attorneys and city merchants. Premiums grew as prospects of profitable medical practice increased by the early nineteenth century, so that John Keats's premium in 1810 was £210 for five years when bound, aged fourteen, to an Edmonton surgeon-apothecary. In the provinces premiums could range from £20 to £84, although £60 or £63 was most commonly recorded. When a youth was indentured to a master who held an honorary hospital post, of which there were increasing numbers by the later eighteenth century, the premium was always substantially more than to a man engaged only in private practice, so that Edward Goldwire, a surgeon at Salisbury Infirmary, took premiums of £210 in the 1750s. By the early nineteenth century, John Green Crosse, an established Norfolk practitioner, with a hospital appointment, was able to note that four apprentices lived in his family house at £100 a year each and that his 'vacancies (were) always pre-engaged'. He himself had been apprenticed in 1806 for five years to a local practitioner with a premium of £200. A provincial surgeon with a good practice could, however, attract far larger premiums than had been paid when he himself was apprenticed; thus Robert Mynors, for whom £50 had been paid, received £157 with each of the eleven youths he indentured in Birmingham, while in 1834 Sir Astley Cooper of Guy's Hospital commented on the very large sums paid in London. Premiums were not paid when a son was apprenticed to his own father.

The details of a medical apprentice's life are largely unrecorded, although some youths kept diaries and noted the tasks they undertook, the skills they acquired and the patients they saw. Many were critical of the experience, especially at the beginning of the term when they had to perform the most humble tasks, cleaning equipment and sweeping floors, so that a prosperous London Quaker apprentice, William Lucas, with a premium of £200 in the 1820s, constantly bemoaned his miserable and physically uncomfortable life. At the lower end of medical apprenticeship, George Crabbe, the poet, working in the 1770s, resented having to walk seven miles to deliver medicines to a patient. As late as 1834 the Select Committee on Medical Education heard how a surgeon-apothecary's apprentice had to answer the door, take messages and make up medicines, while Roderick Random, Smollett's hero, was able to 'bleed and give a clyster, spread a plaister and prepare a potion'. We know from the diary of Richard Kay of Baldingstone, near Bury, trained by his father in the 1740s, that he was allowed to attend patients on his own and often left in charge of the surgery while his father visited the sick at home. John Green Crosse noted that he rolled pills, kept the books and tended the leeches, as well as tidying the surgery. He also wrote extensive case notes all his life. Since apprenticeship was essentially a practical training, accompanying a master on his rounds was vital and the young Henry Jephson, later MD, but bound to a Nottinghamshire parish surgeon in 1812, wrote home in delight to his parents:

> I can with just pleasure add that he behaved like a Gent and has promised to let me visit them alone. I assure you it has happened exactly right in my last year, as I can visit them more than I did before, indeed he advised me to pay attention to the various diseases I see, and you may depend upon my taking it.

Having survived his apprenticeship, a young tradesman would become a jour-neyman, while in medicine he would receive a salary to work as an assistant for a practitioner, join another man as his partner, with shared profits, or set up in practice on his own. A minority were pupils to hospital consultants in London and in the provinces. In all parts of the country there was a strong familial pattern in practice and many medical dynasties, such as the Langfords of Hereford or the Brees of Warwickshire, became prominent in the eighteenth century and were to last until the present. Marrying his master's daughter was an established means of advancing a young man's professional career, and Crosse was but one new practitioner to do so. A wife from a medical household was a considerable asset and the master, perhaps providing a smaller dowry, gained a young partner, trained in his methods, who knew the patients and would keep the practice thriving as he grew older. The master's professional secrets, espe-cially his remedies, would be in safe hands and the newly-qualified young man would neither set up in competition nor join a rival practitioner. Additional capital could be produced for the master by selling practice goodwill to an incoming partner. The master was unlikely, however, to be able to sell practice goodwill to his son-in-law, who would usually join without payment. By having lived in the master's house, the apprentice gained a thorough understanding of practice life – especially important if he came from a non-medical family – the erratic work hours, how to deal with patients, keep case-notes and other records, assess the urgency of calls and plan a round of visits, charging accordingly. He watched his master buy, stock and dispense drugs, judging how to apply a scale of fees according to the patient's prosperity and how to negotiate for parish Poor Law work and for other institutional appointments. He also learned how to supervise apprentices and lay staff, groom, coachman or servant, none of which practical skills was described in contemporary apprenticeship manuals or medical text-books.

Setting up in practice was a critical step for surgeon-apothecaries and, as the 1783 *Medical Register* indicates, few men were in partnerships. In that year there were sixty-two two-man family partnerships listed (5.2 per cent), often with the younger practitioner better qualified than the senior, as well as eighty-eight part-nerships (6.8 per cent) between men of different names, although perhaps linked by marriage or a former master-apprentice relationship. However, the great majority of surgeon-apothecaries, 88 per cent, worked on their own in 1783. Physicians were always in single-handed practice and the views of Erasmus Darwin MD on setting up in practice mirrored his own experiences. He suggested that the young practitioner should use all means to 'get acquainted with people of all ranks', decorate his shop window attractively and appear in public at the farmers' ordinary (public dinner) on market days, at card assemblies and at dances. He also advised letters of introduction and 'dressing to appear well; which money cannot be better laid out'. Erasmus Darwin himself had made several moves to improve his own career, which began in Nottingham, twelve miles from his family home, in 1756 after having qualified at Edinburgh. As his practice did not prosper, he moved a year later to Lichfield and gained an influential patient who introduced Darwin to the midland scientific community. He was prepared to move again in 1781 to Derby, for his second wife preferred her estate at Radbourne to living in Lichfield, and in addition a leading physician had just left Derby to live in London. When Darwin's physician son, Robert, set up in practice in 1786 at Shrewsbury the town had three senior physicians, but Erasmus was able to boast that, as 'a great encouragement', within the first six months the young man had fifty patients, who might conceivably have been attracted to a practitioner with such a distinguished medical name. Clearly, becoming established in practice was the most difficult period for a practitioner, and Christian Esberger confided to his journal for 1764 his doubts about his unsuccessful practice in Lincolnshire; in July he found 'a considerable decay in my accounts; passed it off in hopes of better times to come'. By December he noted 'I have at present hardly any patients, not one of any Significancy to confine me' and considered moving to a nearby town where the apothecary was leaving; he never became a wealthy man.

An important step in the professionalisation of medicine was the publication of medical registers from 1779, enabling patients to choose practitioners and practitioners to contact each other. Surgeons and apothecaries had always been listed in earlier trade directories among others who provided a service, but in 1779 Samuel Foart Simmons, a London physician, published his first *Medical Register*. The *Law List* was not to appear until 1839 and *Crockford's Clerical Directory* until 1870. Simmons's *Register* was arranged on a county basis, and covered the British Isles and overseas, with a strong emphasis on the professional bodies controlling the practitioners. Simmons began by using local contacts to provide the county information, which was arranged alphabetically town by town. He noted if there were a county hospital and sometimes the existence of an asylum or dispensary. A second edition, little improved, appeared a year later but in 1783 he published the third and fullest edition, with much more detail and filling in many of the gaps of earlier versions. It is a remarkable publication, telling the reader where physicians qualified, hospital appointments held and some practitioners' recent moves or deaths.

The 1783 register shows a striking imbalance between the different categories of men and their uneven national coverage. There were 3120 practitioners listed; the unqualified, such as barber-surgeons and bone-setters, were omitted. Of these, 363 were physicians (11.6 per cent), 2,614 were surgeon-apothecaries (83.6 per cent), with 79 apothecaries (2.5 per cent) and 64 surgeons (2.05 per cent). The physicians were concentrated in county towns, often linked to hospitals, in spas and in cathedral cities, for clerics were always particularly good patients, and, even if they were a small community, such as Wells, physicians could join an educated, congenial social group. Physicians were noticeably absent from the developing northern industrial towns but could often be found living near royal residences (Windsor, Hampton Court) or aristocratic seats (Alnwick, Castle Howard). Some spa towns, such as Brighton and Buxton, had physicians only during the season, although Bath uniquely could support fourteen permanent physicians in 1783. All practitioners lived on local road networks, to facilitate contact with their patients, for both physicians and surgeon-apothecaries travelled many miles to visit sufferers at home, presumably not always as comfortably as Erasmus Darwin in his specially-fitted coach.

Surgeon-apothecaries, the majority of practitioners, however, could be found in all areas, usually in market towns, generally in single-handed practice. Where to practise was clearly a business decision and some men can be seen moving to improve their clientèle, to avoid competition or to where a new hospital had opened. Indeed, the coming of county hospitals in provincial England in the second half of the eighteenth century made well over a hundred new career openings possible. Seven were established in the 1740s alone, twenty-nine in the whole century. A hospital definitely attracted aspiring practitioners, who would move to gain an appointment; thus John Storer (MD, Glasgow, 1771), one of three physicians in Grantham in 1783, moved to be the most junior of three physicians at the new Nottingham hospital, opened in 1782, gaining a considerable reputation in the county and practising there well into the next century. Each county infirmary had two to four physicians and the same number of surgeons and an apothecary; there were also posts at the increasing number of dispensaries that were being set up. Such institutions represented a substantial career step for the ambitious practitioner, as the efforts to secure a post in 1810 at the new Derby Infirmary by one young man, Henry Ward, reveal. Having trained in London (Figure 1.1), he had excellent medical references and he also wrote to local men of influence soliciting their support; he was clearly disappointed to fail. The calibre of candidates was such that one of his rivals, equally unsuccessful, for the most junior post in the hospital, that of salaried apothecary, was Henry Lilley Smith, later the founder of Self-Supporting Dispensaries. Ward subsequently practised in north Warwickshire for the rest of his life. John Green Crosse struggled for two years to gain an assistant surgery appointment at Norwich Hospital. Not all practitioners were fulfilled or happy in their careers, but a change of profession was not easy to achieve. We know from their memoirs that George Crabbe, always at the unprosperous end of practice, gave up medicine to enter the church, while John Taylor detested his apprenticeship in Bolton in 1825 and left to study law, later to become a coroner. Some practitioners, however, were able to leave medicine on inheriting or marrying money. Thus John Matthews MD, fourth physician at St George's Hospital, London, became a country gentleman in 1784 when he inherited a family estate in Herefordshire, later an MP and Colonel of the county militia. As well as his medical income, John Johnstone MD inherited a Dumfriesshire estate on the death of his father and became Laird of Galabank in 1774, although continuing to practise. John Simpson MD loathed the constant competition for patients in Bradford in 1825 and wished to increase his private income to £300 a year so that he could retire from practice. His problems were solved with the death of his uncle, a prosperous physician at Malton, whose heir he was, and finally by his marrying a very wealthy heiress.

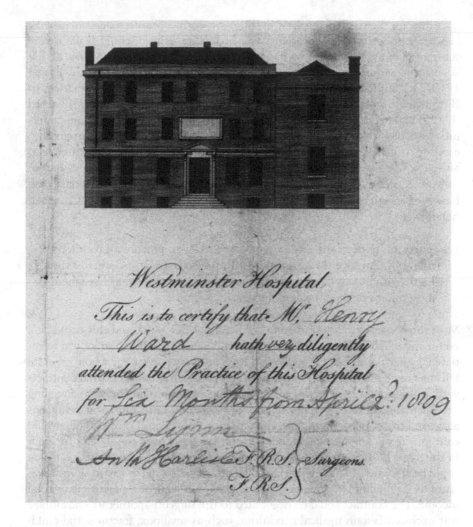

Figure 1.1 Henry Ward's certificate of attendance at Westminster Hospital, signed by William Lynn and Anthony Carlisle. By kind permission of Mr John Driver.

The whole question of medical incomes is problematic largely for lack of reliable evidence. Sometimes practitioners noted earnings in their journals and, for a few, account ledgers and bills have survived. Crosse's private practice brought him £3,500 a year but at the peak of his career Sir Astley Cooper was said to earn £21,000 annually. Cooper also, however, recorded his own annual income for nine years (1792–1800) before he was appointed as a surgeon at Guy's Hospital. It increased strikingly from £5 5s. in 1792 to £100 by 1796 and to £1,100 by 1800. By 1813 he could charge a wealthy merchant a thousand guineas when operating for the stone. Even early in the eighteenth century a successful provincial practitioner, with élite patients and little competition, could make a very substantial living in practice, as illustrated in the papers of Claver Morris MD of Wells, who earned nearly £300 a year attending some 250 patients in the period 1718–21. William Small MD made £500 a year from town practice in Birmingham, which rose to £600 by the 1770s, while Samuel Malins MD noted that his highest annual income of £525 17s. 6d. in Liverpool, largely from maternity work, was achieved in 1841. However, an undistinguished surgeon-apothecary, in a rural practice, could make a comfortable living of some £150 a year; although a perpetual problem for such practitioners remained patients who were slow to settle their accounts, this mattered little in a non-inflationary age. However, shortly after the Barbers' and Surgeons' Company had split, Campbell noted that:

> There are none of the Liberal Arts more likely to procure a Livelihood than this. An ingenious Surgeon, let him be cast on any Corner of the Earth, with but his Case of Instruments in his Pocket, he may live where most other Professions would starve.

Most surgeon-apothecaries would undertake Poor Law work and this could be a useful and reliable source of income, especially when a parish contract was negotiated, rather than charging individual fees for every pauper, for whom separate bills had to be submitted. Undoubtedly, Overseers of the Poor preferred contracts with a surgeon, for they gained his services for a known annual charge, avoiding the fluctuations caused by epidemics or an increased birth rate. Some surgeons also liked this form of a guaranteed annual income, certain of what they would earn for the year. When Sir Frederic Morton Eden surveyed the state of the poor in the mid-1790s he often noted the parish surgeon's annual contract rate, which could be as low as £10 at Petersfield and Lancaster or as high as £30 in Warrington and £54 in Bradford, although such fees were only part of a practitioner's total income. The contract could be negotiated to the surgeon-apothecary's advantage if it excluded certain medical conditions, such as smallpox, fractures and childbirth, for which extra charges were made. Some practitioners were hardly prosperous, however, and the career of Gideon Mantell in the early nineteenth century, as he struggled to be paid and also to purchase a practice (in instalments of £95 a year for seven years), illustrates how difficult it could be to make a living from medical practice.

Occasionally, the obituary notice of a very successful practitioner noted his wealth, so that William Lewis of Oxford left a fortune of £35,000 in 1772 gained 'by his extensive practice'. Eminent men such as William Hunter and Richard Mead were actually, not merely reputedly, very rich from practice and the constant complaints from patients about their large medical bills explains how these men prospered. The successful practitioner could be easily assessed in contemporary society by his general lifestyle, particularly his house, carriage, acquaintances and clientèle. Apart from a house with a good address, a physician's setting up costs were moderate; he needed a library, consulting room, some form of transport and the usual domestic servants. Some professional premises, long used for medical practice, had valuable goodwill attached to them, so that, for example, Tobias Smollett MD moved into John Douglas's house in Downing Street, London in 1744 and John Blount practised in the 1780s from a house in Temple Row, Birmingham where 'Chesshire the surgeon used to live'. Established medical premises as a part of professional goodwill remained an important factor until the early days of the National Health Service. As he initially had very little income, the young physician often needed his family's support.

Prosperous practitioners were regularly benefactors to local charities and many held high public office. Thus apothecaries James Dodsworth in 1733 and his former apprentice, Thomas Bowes, in 1761 and 1777, both served as Lord Mayor of York, William Dawson was Mayor of Leeds in 1770 and Edward Harper of Coventry in 1778, while others acted as charitable trustees and governors. For many of the grandest practitioners, usually physicians, their portraits survive, often by the best artists (Allan Ramsay's portrait of William Hunter, Joshua Reynolds's of John Ash and of Percival Pott, Roubiliac's bust of Richard Mead). At their death, they were frequently given imposing monuments (Figure 1.2) and fulsome obituary notices:

> YORK, March 15 (1748)
> Last Saturday died Dr Wintringham, a very eminent Physician of this City. A Gentleman so universally known and esteem'd, for his extensive Knowledge in his Profession, both in this City and County, that to give him a longer Character would be here needless.

Apart from their years at university or as apprentices, quite a substantial minority of young men went on to be trained in hospitals, although sometimes only briefly, taking one or two courses and usually not to hold hospital appointments themselves. Except for the great naval hospitals, infirmary appointments for physicians and surgeons were honorary, so those holding such posts were personally able to charge considerable pupil fees to offset their unpaid service. Pupils, apprentices and dressers, attached to a leading hospital consultant after finishing an apprenticeship, paid substantial sums for the privilege, while less prosperous pupils simply 'walked the wards' as observers. The range of practical tuition a young man might receive was vividly noted in the diary of William Shippen, an American who spent a year in London in 1759:

> 30 July went thro the hospital by myself to examine the patients ... spent 2 hours in examining a dead body at hospital who died suddenly ... 4 August saw Mr Way surgeon to Guy's hospital amputate a leg above the knee very dexterously 3 ligatures ... 23 August attended Dr

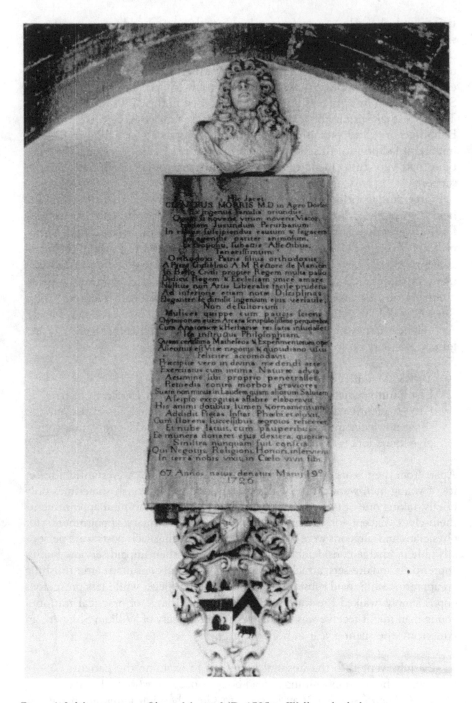

Figure 1.2 Monument to Claver Morris, MD, 1725 in Wells cathedral.

Akenside in taking in patients and prescribing for them, 56 taken in ...
5 September examined particulars in hospital several small pox 3 out of
4 die, saw Mr. Baker perform 3 operations, a leg, breast and tumour from
a girl's lower jaw inside, very well operated. Mr. Warner extracted a
large stone from urethra of a man and pinn'd the incision up as in a
harelip ... 2 November went to Georges Hospital and saw Hawkins and
Bromfield operate, stone and amputation ... 7 November went to
Bartholomews Hospital and saw the neatest operation of bubonocele
that ever I saw by Mr. Pott a very clever neat surgeon.

As well as pupil fees, various examination and other expenses were incurred as a
medical student; one young man in only six months (1828–9) noted spending
£130 3s. 6d., including his apothecary's certificate, on his London training, apart
from books, equipment and dissection specimens on which to practise his skills.
In his evidence to the 1834 Select Committee on Medical Education, Sir Astley
Cooper, an anatomy lecturer at St Thomas's and a consultant at Guy's Hospital,
described the three classes of students in London hospitals. These were the
apprentice, who paid £500 or £600 and lived in the surgeon's own home, the
dresser, who paid '£500 for the privilege of dressing for 12 months' and the pupil,
who paid £26 5s. for a year's tuition. Lecture charges were added to these fees and
also the costs of dissection and courses in *materia medica* and physiology. Cooper
recalled that he had himself lived with Henry Cline as a pupil and had attended
John Hunter's lectures. He had formerly been apprenticed in 1784 with a
premium of £535 for seven years. He also described how hard he worked while
still a hospital pupil:

> I went to the hospital before breakfast to dissect for lecture. I demon-
> strated to the students before lecture. I injected their subjects. I lectured
> from two o'clock till half-past three. In the evening, three times per
> week, I lectured on surgery. I attended to the interesting cases in the
> hospital, making notes of them, and in the latter practice I always per-
> severed.

It has long been argued that honorary hospital posts were accepted because the
practitioners were thus in good standing with the local gentry and aristocracy,
the infirmary's benefactors and governors, who might later become lucrative
patients. There was also the free publicity to be gained as honorary staff when
the annual infirmary reports were distributed, since the names of the physicians
and surgeons were always prominent on the front page. The professional desire
to specialise must also have motivated some men to serve, as well as the
Christian's duty to sufferers, a motive largely under-valued by modern
researchers.

However, the efforts many eminent men made to secure hospital appointments
suggest that an infirmary post was widely well-regarded in a locality, whatever the

individual's motives. The 1834 Select Committee commented adversely on the degree of nepotism in hospital posts and, although this view was challenged, substantial evidence exists to support the criticism, for Astley Cooper himself had five relatives in posts at St Thomas's and Guy's Hospitals and received £3,000 a year from their students. In the provinces the Johnstone family – James, Edward and John – shared out infirmary appointments in Worcester and Birmingham in the eighteenth century, while the university link was always a strong one in patronage terms, so that in the eighteenth century all physicians at Manchester Hospital were Edinburgh men, as were those at Lincoln and Birmingham.

It is clear that, from at least the mid-eighteenth century, the growing population's use of all practitioners increased considerably as medical skills widened to include new techniques (such as inoculation), surgical procedures (couching for cataract), and as more effective drugs became available. There were also, for some men, fresh career opportunities in obstetric work, as the traditional midwife's services were superseded in prosperous families by those of an *accoucheur* or man-midwife. Perhaps the most striking aspect of eighteenth-century medical practice, however, particularly for surgeon-apothecaries, was the range of new semi-official work that became available across the country. Apart from Poor Law, prison, asylum, infirmary and dispensary posts, which expanded substantially, practitioners were increasingly required to examine apprentices going to factories, men joining the militia, prisoners in gaols and felons being transported, providing expert evidence in court as well as inspecting madhouses and factories. All friendly societies, whose numbers swelled in Georgian England (see Chapter 4), needed practitioners to examine, treat and certify sick members. Although Foart Simmons noted only eight dispensaries in 1783, all attended by physicians, their numbers were to grow most noticeably of all institutions after 1800 (see Chapter 5). As the eighteenth century was one of almost continuous warfare for Britain, more military and naval appointments were available to which men could move from civilian practice, and the 1783 *Register* illustrates that a substantial number of practitioners had served in the army or navy, if only for a short period.

An important area of growth for a minority of entrepreneurial practitioners, both physicians and surgeon-apothecaries, was the development of private lunatic asylums, either because there were genuinely more patients to be admitted or because contemporary definitions of madness changed to include categories of inmates it was not formerly thought necessary to incarcerate (see Chapter 6). Although many were run by lay proprietors, those most highly regarded by contemporaries, and the most expensive, were owned and supervised by qualified practitioners. Simmons in 1783 noted only five provincial asylums run by physicians, Nathaniel Cotton at St Albans, Thomas Arnold at Leicester, Francis Willis at Stamford, William Perfect at Malling and John Beevor at Norwich. There were also posts for physicians at the public institutions for the insane at Newcastle upon Tyne, Norwich and York. Simmons did not mention the asylums run by surgeon-apothecaries, such as those at Henley-in-Arden, Hook Norton or Bilston, nor those run by medically unqualified lay proprietors. The exceptional entrepreneur, such as Richard Wilkes MD of Willenhall, though too early to be listed by Simmons, had promoted a 'Spaw' on his land in the 1740s, which must have found favour with sufferers because of its medical connections.

From a comparison of medical lists across the later eighteenth and early nineteenth centuries, it is obvious that the numbers of practitioners, at all levels, were growing. Birmingham provides a good example of such professional growth for, although its economic expansion during this period was remarkable, it was echoed in many great northern cities and everywhere by 1850 there were many more practitioners than there had been in 1750. In Birmingham the increase was fivefold.

Table 1.1   Medical practitioners in Birmingham, 1767–1850

Year	Surgeons	Physicians	Population	Population/practitioners ratio
1767	20	3	23,688 in 1750	10,299 : 1
1783	19	4	52,250 in 1785	2271 : 1
1792	37	8	60,822 in 1801	1351 : 1
1811	39	6	70,207 in 1811	1560 : 1
1818	43	6	85,416 in 1821	1743 : 1
1828	64	9	110,914 in 1831	1519 : 1
1850	109	15	173,951 in 1851	1402 : 1

Throughout the eighteenth and nineteenth centuries, a surprising number of practitioners were authors, both on medical and other topics. Physicians as authors might be expected, educated men with élite patients, and many indeed were well-known and prolific medical writers, such as Richard Mead. However, other relatively unknown practitioners, both physicians and surgeon-apothecaries, turned their observations and case-notes into publications. Certainly authorship was a means of being recognised and for some, anxious to advance their careers, this must have been a strong motive. Simmons noted medical publications, and often MD dissertation topics, in the 1779 Register but had discontinued doing so by 1783, presumably because the list would have been very lengthy indeed. However, not all medical publications were for other practitioners, for many were widely advertised in the contemporary press and bought by a lay readership, as can be seen from the number of copies in gentlemen's libraries. Some men wrote on scientific but non-medical topics, such as cattle plague (Richard Wilkes in 1743), while The Gouty Man's Companion (1747) by John Cheshire MB was clearly intended as an advice manual for a lay readership. It is obvious, however, that works based on personal experience, such as William Withering's Account of the Foxglove (1785), largely a series of case-notes and other practitioners' views, were meant for professional colleagues, as were Robert Mynors's accounts of amputation (1783) and trepanning (1785), Jonathan Stokes's Botanical Materia Medica, Richard Wilkes on dropsy (1730) and smallpox (1747), John Green Crosse's publication in 1851 of his own 1,377 midwifery cases or Hugh Owen Thomas's *Diseases of the Hip, Knee and Ankle Joints with their Deformities* (1875).

Sometimes a medical publication was meant to influence a wider readership than the purely professional. Thus Thomas Tomlinson, a shadowy provincial surgeon-man-midwife, but with wide clinical experience at both Birmingham workhouse and the General Hospital, published his *Medical Miscellany* in 1769, with a second edition five years later. He dedicated the book to Caesar Hawkins, the London surgeon. As well as his views on medical education, Tomlinson wrote in uncompromising terms about the diseases of the poor and the occupational health of the area, of which he had considerable first-hand experience, presumably hoping to interest local men of influence. Indeed, occupational disease was one medical area in which wider polemical texts can be found, with Charles Turner Thackrah's *The Effects of the Principal Arts, Trades and Professions…on Health and Longevity* of 1832 following in an honourable tradition that began with Bernard Ramazzini more than a century earlier, addressed as much to employers and workers as to practitioners.

A number of practitioners, especially genteel physicians, had keen antiquarian interests. Thus Richard Wilkes of Staffordshire recorded archaeological discoveries and was involved with Stebbing Shaw's plan for a history of his county, while John Johnstone prepared the Kidderminster section for T. R. Nash's *History of Worcestershire* (1781–2). Simmons noted that William Pryce MD of Redruth was publishing a book on the ancient Cornish language, while one of the earliest eighteenth-century local historians, Francis Drake, was a surgeon-apothecary of York and author of *Eboracum* (1736); John Burton MD, who practised in the same city, wrote *Monasticon Eboranse* twenty years later. The Society of Antiquaries of London, founded in 1717, had a noticeable number of medical members and its first secretary was a practitioner, William Stukeley MD. In the early nineteenth century, Gideon Mantell seemed discontented in medical practice and really happy only when collecting geological specimens, his true vocation, noting how he had 'muddled away another week doing nothing. The same dull round of visiting patients'. Geology was in fact a fashionable interest shared by William Small and Henry Jephson. Some practitioners, such as Jonathan Stokes of Chesterfield, were eminent in other scientific fields, publishing his four-volume *Botanical commentaries*, the standard work, in 1830. There were of course, in addition, practitioners who were really writers, for example, George Crabbe or Erasmus Darwin, and are remembered as such rather than as surgeons or physicians.

A number of practitioners had unusual, even bizarre, interests and obsessions, so that Jonathan Stokes promoted a reformed orthography, using no double letters or apostrophes and with few capitals, while Henry Lilley Smith sought to prove the accuracy of the Apocalypse. Others, however, although ordinary provincial practitioners, made practical scientific contributions to medicine, so that Richard Pearson introduced *lichen Islandicus* as a cure for indigestion, Robert Mynors devised a many-tailed bandage for amputation stumps and John Burton invented a new-style forceps. The very grandest men were also collectors and patrons of the arts, with William Hunter, Richard Mead and, earlier, Sir Hans Sloane all distinguished in this field. On a more modest scale, some practitioners had botanical gardens and collections, such as John Fothergill's garden at Upton, John Blackburne's at Orford Hall, near Warrington in the 1780s or Jonathan Stokes's herbarium in Derbyshire early in the next century. Many practitioners were involved in non-medical philanthropy, presumably as a result of their professional experience, so that the Quaker, Lettsom, was interested in such welfare schemes as relieving small debtors, preventing drowning, educating the deaf and dumb and employing the blind.

It is impossible to estimate how many practitioners in the eighteenth century belonged to scientific and medical societies, for few such organisations have good surviving records. Simmons noted the Literary and Philosophical Societies at Leeds, Liverpool and Manchester, dominated by medical practitioners, as well as the Medical Society founded at Colchester in 1774, the only provincial society so named, to which three physicians and sixteen surgeon-apothecaries belonged. By the end of the century, however, there were many more similar societies established, as at Bath, Bristol, Reading, Donnington and Spalding. Simmons also noted a Botanical Society recently founded at Lichfield, even though it never had more than three members. Chester and Liverpool had Inoculation Societies, while there were Humane Societies on the London model at both Leeds and Liverpool. The Derby Philosophical Society, founded in 1783, had fifty-two members in its first twenty years, of whom eleven were surgeons and fifteen were other practitioners, including physicians. The century's most prestigious scientific group, the Lunar Society of Birmingham, established in 1765, had only fourteen members, of whom four were physicians (Darwin, Small, Stokes and Withering), and was clearly a group for only the most eminent, amongst whom the newly-qualified would not have been acceptable or at ease. Some men belonged to several societies, so that John Johnstone joined the groups at Manchester and Bath as well as the London and Edinburgh Medical Societies. Stokes was also one of the first sixteen Associates of the Linnean Society in 1790, having met Linnaeus earlier when plant-collecting in Europe. After the Provincial Medical and Surgical Association, later to become the British Medical Association, was founded at Worcester in 1832, its meetings were held in various regions enabling many more practitioners to enjoy the benefits of a professional membership. Thus in 1834 John Green Crosse went to its meeting at Oxford to hear the founder, Charles Hastings, speak and then he himself set up the Eastern branch. All such organisations must have considerably helped to form the idea of a cohesive profession and to expand practitioners' contacts, which had been almost entirely personal earlier in the century. From their letters, however, we know that even the provincial practitioner might have links with the wider scientific world, so that John Johnstone in Worcestershire corresponded with Baron Haller, William Small in Birmingham with Joseph Priestley and Jonathan Stokes in Derbyshire with Sir Joseph Banks, L'Heritier and Solander.

Until the nineteenth century, the training of practitioners in hospitals varied greatly from one institution to another and was essentially controlled by the senior men in the hospital as to syllabus, length of courses, fees and practical experience. Hospital training was essentially an option for the élite student, not compulsory and certainly not required to engage in practice. Although the Select Committee on Medical Education revealed the main outlines of training for the 1830s, very few first-hand accounts have survived of hospital training from an earlier period. As part of a hospital pupil's training was to record what cases and demonstrations he had seen, it might be expected that such accounts would survive in considerable numbers. They are, however, archivally scarce and only one of Keats's notebooks has survived, for example. Richard Kay wrote briefly of his London hospital training at St Thomas's and Guy's, learning dissection from William Sharpe and John Girle, as well as midwifery from William Smellie, while William Shippen in 1759 recorded surgeons he had seen at work. However, the occasional very rare survival, such as the student lecture notes kept by Thomas Woen Jones in 1796, suggests that originally these may well have been written by all conscientious hospital pupils as a reference source to be consulted when the pupil was later in practice on his own far from his teachers. Jones's extensive notes refer to midwifery cases. He was taught by William Osborne MD, physician at the New Lying-In Hospital in Store Street, the author of two textbooks on difficult labours and responsible for a design to improve the obstetric forceps; Osborne claimed to have taught midwifery to over 1,200 students. Jones's other lecturer was John Clarke MD, who had also written two books on pregnancy and taught midwifery at St Bartholomew's. However, in 1790, Jones's year in London, he also noted the views of eight other leading practitioners, including William Bromfield, William Fordyce and William Hunter; his lecture notes included such topics as 'Management of the Placenta', 'Diseases of Women' and 'Problems of inversion, flooding and lochial discharge'. Jones then practised in Warwickshire, chiefly in midwifery, for fifty years. It is clear, however, that being taught by a highly distinguished man encouraged students to keep their casenotes and some dozen sets have survived from those written by John Hunter's many students.

Undoubtedly, medicine had become more socially acceptable, even genteel, by the early nineteenth century, although still below the law and the church in perceived status. Clearly, a major problem for medicine in gaining acceptance as a career for gentlemen was public revulsion at dissection, noted by a foreign visitor in 1791:

> The aversion of the English to anatomical dissections is another of the prejudices which characterize that nation. The surgeons have great difficulty in procuring dead bodies; they are obliged to pay large sums for them, and are forced to carry them to their houses with utmost secrecy. If the people hear of it, they assemble in crowds around the house, and break the windows.

This was particularly because the illegal means of acquiring cadavers before the passing of the Anatomy Act in 1831 aroused widespread horror and disgust. Dissection, however, was the acknowledged means of gaining knowledge and greater skills for the twin disciplines of anatomy and surgery. Bichat indeed advised his students when they experienced difficulty in diagnosis, 'Open up a few corpses: you will dissipate at once the darkness that observation alone could not dispel'.

The Barber Surgeons' Company in 1530 had been granted (22 Henry VIII, c.12) the bodies of four malefactors a year, taken from the gallows, for public post mortem examination; the number was increased to six by Charles II. Thus dissection came to be seen as an aggravated punishment in addition to a death sentence, particularly when, in 1752, an Act was passed to allow dissection instead of gibbeting for particularly heinous offences. Thus when Broughton and Hayes were executed at Tyburn for rioting in 1752, their bodies went to John Harrison, founding surgeon at the London Hospital, to be publicly dissected 'as a Terror to other offenders in such atrocious crimes'. Unfortunately, William Hunter's scheme for a school and museum of anatomy was rejected by the government and the strong criminal links with dissection became increasingly common for nearly a century. Hunter was also obliged to use illegally acquired corpses, as graphically described in one London newspaper in 1783 when a body was delivered to a shocked housekeeper at the front door of the physician's house.

Private anatomy schools had existed in London from at least the early eighteenth century and, although their courses of lectures were widely advertised in the press (twenty-seven have been traced), no mention was ever made that dissection was actually carried out. William Hunter, for example, bought an anatomy school at Covent Garden as a going concern in 1764 from William Sharpe (who had taught Richard Kay) and it is clear that Hunter's work would have been impossible without cadavers to dissect. Two years later he established his new premises in Great Windmill Street, which became the country's most famous anatomy school, continued by Matthew Baillie after Hunter's death in 1783. Hunter in fact seems to have delivered 112 lectures over a period of fourteen weeks for a student's fee of £7 7s. and he frequently had a hundred students. In 1775 the course comprised two introductory lectures, fifteen on operative surgery, eighty on anatomy, twelve on midwifery and three on making 'preparations' and embalming. Only chemistry and *materia medica* were to be acquired elsewhere. He claimed to teach 'in the French manner', a code for dissecting cadavers, and the eminent George Fordyce recalled that he had dissected three as a Hunter pupil. However, Hunter warned his students against talking of their anatomical work with him for fear of public disquiet. The term 'practical anatomy', clearly implying dissection, was not noted as a feature of anatomy courses in the London hospitals until 1802. Shocking stories about body-snatching regularly appeared in the contemporary press:

10 January 1784: On Tuesday the 23 of December last, Mr. S., professor of anatomy, Great Queen-street, employed a man to procure him a dead body, that he might demonstrate the muscels the day following to his young pupils, amounting to upwards of seventy. The man according to agreement brought the body in a sack the same evening to his dissecting room, but shocking to relate, on examining the body, he found it to be his own sister, that was buried at Kensington on the 14th, the sight of which threw Mr. S. into strong convulsions, and he now lies dangerously ill.

Mr S. was, in fact, John Sheldon, MRCS, FRS, who lectured at his house in Great Queen Street, served as surgeon at the General Medical Asylum and was Professor of Anatomy at the Royal Academy; he did not die until 1808 at the age of fifty-four.

The whole question of supplying bodies for dissection was clearly kept as secret as possible. In law, if resurrectionists stole nothing but the corpse, not clothing or the coffin, they could really be charged only with trespassing, while the surgeons who commissioned the grave-robbers and paid for the bodies were not punished. Accounts of grave-robbing appeared regularly in the eighteenth-century press and, to protect a recent burial, watchers could be hired to guard the site until the body was too decomposed to be of value for post mortem dissection. An alternative was to put a large iron cage, called a mortsafe, or railings to protect the burial plot or to use an iron coffin, which was noisy to exhume.

Corpses were particularly required by medical students, who were often less than sensitive in their behaviour; thus George Crabbe's landlady found a dead child in his closet while another young hospital pupil took home amputated limbs from the Birmingham workhouse on which to practise his dissecting skills. In his cash book for 1829, one young perpetual pupil, taught by Cooper and Abernethy, noted buying four specimens, preserved and injected, a leg, head, neck and abdomen, costing 18s. 3d. each. The need was greatest, however, for hospitals with medical schools; there was, for example, a six-fold increase of students at St Thomas's Hospital at this period. Bodies were often moved many miles to meet this demand; London corpses were despatched to Manchester, Birmingham, Bristol and Exeter, while Liverpool sent bodies to Edinburgh and Glasgow. In early nineteenth-century York there was a spate of grave-robbing by a well-organised gang to supply the anatomy departments in Edinburgh, with a direct coaching route between the cities. The surgeons would pay quite substantial prices for bodies and pass these charges on to their students, even forming themselves into an Anatomical Club to regulate prices in their dealings with the resurrectionists. A remarkable survival in the form of a resurrectionist's working diary has survived for the year 1811–12, kept by Joseph Naples, a former grave-digger, who worked with a team of eight men supplying the leading London hospitals with corpses, often bribing the local churchyard keepers and usually robbing several graves in any one night. Naples's distinguished customers included John Taunton, principal lecturer to the London Anatomical Society, Henry Cline, anatomical lecturer at St Thomas's, Joseph Carpue, founder of the Dean Street Anatomical School, Algernon Frampton, physician at the London Hospital, James Wilson of the Great Windmill Street School, Joshua Brookes, founder of the Blenheim Street Anatomical School, Astley Cooper, anatomical lecturer at St Thomas's and Sir Charles Bell, Professor of Surgery at Edinburgh. Cooper later left instructions for his own post mortem to be carried out at his death in 1841 and for the results to be published. In the resurrectionist market-place, an adult corpse cost at least £4 4s., although £7 17s. 6d. was once recorded, and bodies were graded as large, small and 'foetus'. During this one year, Naples noted receipts totalling £1,394 8s. He continued his activities until the passing of the Anatomy Act twenty years later, when he worked as a servant in the dissecting room of St Thomas's Hospital. One of his associates, Jack Harnett, was said to have died worth nearly £6,000.

It was undoubtedly the activities and notoriety of Burke and Hare that made action necessary when it was found that they had carried out sixteen murders to provide bodies for dissection. *The Lancet* echoed the findings of the Select Committee on Anatomy (1828) when its editorial thundered, 'It is disgusting to talk of anatomy as a science, whilst it is cultivated by means of practices which would disgrace a nation of cannibals'. The Anatomy Act came into being as a result of the activities of Henry Warburton MP to regulate the supply of bodies to the anatomy schools and became law in December 1831. It was not, however, universally accepted, for the poor objected to its section seven, which authorised parish officers, workhouse masters and hospitals to consign unclaimed pauper bodies to the anatomists. Even after the Act, fears for the safety of corpses, especially among the poor, were still common, so that, for example, in 1839 a rumour was circulating in remote Worcestershire that a recent pauper burial had been disinterred 'and his body recognised in the dissecting room at Birmingham'; the parish Board of Guardians moved swiftly to investigate. Dickens's Jerry Cruncher, some twenty years later, illustrates what a powerful fear body-snatching continued to be in the popular mind, with some justification, for as late as 1858 the master of Newington workhouse was arrested for selling pauper bodies over a ten-year period; he was not convicted, but he was said to have received as much as £26 for each corpse.

There was still, even after the 1834 Select Committee had met, no structured system of medical education in England and only physicians had nationally recognised formal qualifications, the university MD. However, by the middle years of the nineteenth century, reforms were apparent in several areas of medicine. The Apothecaries' Act of 1815 had regularised their branch of medicine and the publication of a medical register required by the 1858 Act was to create a modern profession. Medicine would in future be able to control its own educational standards, examinations and qualifications, separating the qualified from the irregular practitioner. It also implied certain standards in professional behaviour that, if not maintained, could result in a practitioner's name being struck off the register. Registration clearly brought monopoly to medical care and a consequent improvement of status and enhanced income. Medicine also gained greater public regard as it became more scientific, with hospital appointments as the professional peak. Numbers practising medicine also increased, making the profession more powerful, but so did the population, so that whereas in 1840 there were 10.7 practitioners for every 10,000, by 1880 the ratio was 6.6 per 10,000. By then, there was a change in emphasis in medical training, adding the laboratory as an area for learning to the bedside, hospital and autopsy room. In addition, hospitals became more medically controlled, especially the specialised institutions, with benefactors and gentry far less in control than earlier in the century. Hospital capacity also increased considerably in the late Victorian period, so that, for example, St Thomas's out-patient numbers grew tenfold by 1890 from 10,000 in 1880 and while there were some 65,000 beds in all types of hospitals in 1861, this number had nearly doubled to 113,000 by 1891, figures that powerfully reflected the growth and prestige of all kinds of medicine by the twentieth century.

John Hunter's treatment of William Hickey, the diarist, in 1776

(Hickey had badly burned his foot while staying at Margate with a friend, Mr Cane)

...my friend Cane was greatly distressed. He instantly dispatched an express to London to summon Mr Robin Adair* to come and attend me, but that gentleman happening to be at Bristol at the time, Mr. John Hunter, who had undertaken to act for him during his absence, instantly left town and came to me. After meeting the Margate surgeon and inspecting my foot he at once declared no ill consequence would arise, and that a few days' quiet, keeping my leg in a horizontal position, and frequently applying an embrocation which he ordered, would completely cure the hurt. And so it proved; in a week I was perfectly recovered, but during that period I was kept upon chicken broth, and not allowed a drop of wine, lest fever should ensue.

George Qvist, *John Hunter, 1728–1793*, 1981, p. 168

*Robert Adair was Inspector-General of Hospitals; he was succeeded by Hunter in 1790.

The Diary of a Resurrectionist, 1811

Wednesday 4th December At night went out and got 10, whole [all the gang] went to Green and got 4, Black Crib 1, Bunner fields 5.

Thursday 5th December The whole at home all night.

Friday 6th December Removed 1 from Barthol. to Carpue. At night went out and got 8, Danl at home all night. 6 Back St Lukes & 2 Big Gates: went 5 Barthol. 1 Frampton, 3 St Thomas's, 3 Wilson.

Saturday 7th December At night went out & got 3 at Bunhill Row. 1 St Thomas's, 2 Brookes.

Sunday 8th December At home all night.

Monday 9th December At night went out and got 4 Bethnall Green.

Tuesday 10th December intoxsicated all day: at night went out & got 5 Bunhill Row. Jack all most buried.

Wednesday 11 December Tom & Bill and me removed 5 from St Barthol^w, 2 Wilson, 2 Brookes, 1 Bell; in the evening got 1 Harp[er]s, went to St Thomas, at home all night.

Thursday 12th December I went up to Brookes and Wilson, afterwards me Bill and Daniel went to Bethnall Green, got 2; Jack, Ben went got 2 large & 1 small back St Luke's, came home, aferwards met again & went to Bunhill row got 6, 1 of them with [her throat] cut named Mary Rolph, aged 46, Died 5th Dec. 1811.

Friday 13th December At Home all day & night.

Saturday 14th December Went to Bartholomew took^d two Brookes: Pack^d 4 and sent them to Edinborough, came Home to Ben^n, settled £14 6s. 2½d. each man, came home, got up at 2 me Jack & Bill went to Bunhill Row and got 3. Ben & Daniel staid at home.

J. B. Bailey, *The Diary of a Resurrectionist*, 1896, pp. 140–2.

The original diary is at the Royal College of Surgeons of London.

2

POPULATION AND
CONTRACEPTION

Our progressive population must have added to the Number of dependent poor
... but it has been a matter of controversy between very able and learned men,
whether an increase or a decrease of people has been going on in this country
during the present century.

David Davies, *The Case of Labourers in Husbandry*, 1795, p. 53

Although it is easy to recognise that the population of England had grown beyond
all contemporary forecasts during the eighteenth century, the reasons for this
increase have been constantly disputed, for greater life expectancy could have been
caused by men and women living longer, more infants being born to become adults
or a combination of these factors. Survival and good health have always primarily
been class-related and yet infections and accidents could kill even the most prosperous. In the early seventeenth century, although the average life expectancy was
only 38.7 years, the heirs of Jacobean squires and above who reached the age of
twenty-one could hope to survive until 63. The prospect for married females was
noticeably worse, however, even for aristocratic wives, of whom 45 per cent died
before the age of 50 in the years 1558–1641, a quarter from childbirth and its com-
plications. In spite of these figures, Francis Bacon was able to comment in 1623
that he saw at least one person over sixty in every village. In the 1640s the death
rate of one-year-olds was 18 per cent and between 40 and 50 per cent of the population in the Civil War years were below the age of twenty.

Various attempts to count the population were made in the early modern
period and for very different reasons. The Hearth Tax, covering the years
1662–88, recorded only hearths as a taxable means of estimating the size of
household, but matches Gregory King's estimate of an average of 4.5 persons in
each in 1695. The Compton Census of 1676 had counted only those over the age
of sixteen according to their religious persuasion, Anglicans, non-Conformists or
Catholics, while the Marriage Tax assessments of the late 1690s, although
invaluable for noting all the inhabitants of a house and their status/occupation,
have hardly survived for anywhere except the London parishes. However, in the
last thirty years, parish register research, and particularly population reconstitu-

tion, has given us a clearer picture of how many people were born, married and died, even though the causes of fluctuations in mortality are far less clear.

By the eighteenth century, however, the population question was pressing and contemporary governments' anxieties changed from fear that there were too few marriages and births to concern that there were too many for the economy to support. Even if the percentage of poor could remain the same, in a growing population their overall increased numbers required more medical services, including infirmaries and dispensaries, as well as wider inoculation provisions. Between 1781 and 1939 the population of England and Wales rose between five- and six-fold, from 7.5 to 41.5 million, and there is little evidence that medical services expanded in proportion, whether in numbers of medical personnel or institutions, although growth certainly took place. Population increase really only occurred after the mid-eighteenth century and the factors that inhibited expansion before c. 1750 were powerful. The years 1700–50 were a period of almost constant warfare for England, removing men of marriageable age from their families and often killing them; famines during this period were not merely severe but continuous one after the other, giving society no chance to recover in intervening prosperous years. Only after 1750, with the Stuart settlement laws virtually ineffective, was there real social mobility in a thriving economy – thus marriage partners could be found further from home. Not only did earlier marriage encourage a population growth, but enhanced fertility was achieved by an expanding gene pool as young men and women increasingly married outside the parish enclave in which they and their ancestors had lived and interbred for centuries. In addition, the first half of the eighteenth century saw smallpox in its more virulent forms and, although inoculation came to England in 1726 with Lady Mary Wortley Montagu's return from the Middle East, it was not in general use, in the provinces especially, until the 1740s, although by the 1760s parish inoculations of the poor were commonplace (see Chapter 8). Even the partial control of smallpox, however, had a crucial effect on population growth, not only in reducing deaths in the population as a whole, but in preventing adult males from becoming victims, among whom infertility was a common after-effect of the disease in survivors, thereby reducing family sizes in the first half of the century. It is questionable how far medical activity affected the population growth. Certainly after c. 1750 voluntary infirmaries began to appear (nineteen in England by 1800) and there were undoubtedly more practitioners at work across the whole country by the end of the century. However, both developments touched only lightly upon the health of the general mass of the people, for hospitals admitted only few, carefully selected patients and professional fees restricted medical attention, except through the Poor Law. In addition, the reduced virulence of some diseases, such as influenza, over the decades meant that even epidemics were not necessarily the severe check on population that the earlier eighteenth century had experienced.

Contemporary opinion attributed the rising birth rate to growing domestic industry and an enhanced demand for labour, bringing higher wages and a better standard of living, thus encouraging workers to breed. Both Malthus and Arthur Young shared Adam Smith's view

> The reward of labour must necessarily encourage in such a manner the marriage and multiplication of labourers, as may enable them to supply that continually increasing demand by a continually increasing population.

Once the main changes affecting the population growth were in place – fecundity, female age at marriage, a wider field of sexual partners, a better diet and some control of diseases – the restraints were off and England's population increase was to continue inexorably. Even when circumstances were difficult the trend could not be reversed and the population continued to swell in bad harvests, poor trading conditions and land scarcity, when smaller families would undoubtedly have been economically preferable. Equally, the population must have been producing survivors, those with some natural immunity to infectious diseases. The simple fact that women were marrying earlier by the mid-eighteenth century, at twenty-one instead of, on average, at twenty-four, meant the possibility of two or three more pregnancies in the three years. In addition, after 1747 male apprentices' terms ended at twenty-one rather than, as before, at twenty-four, legally allowing and encouraging earlier marriages, a generally unappreciated factor in the population debate. Adam Smith's opinion that families increased because of the labour economy presupposed that in some way parents might be able to control their fertility and births. This was clearly not so, except by celibacy, for all the contemporary methods of contraception were ineffective and it was the high death rate among the newly-born that dramatically limited family size. Once this changed, the population inevitably increased. During the years 1730–1809 the infant death rate fell noticeably; in 1730–49 it was 74.5 deaths per hundred live births, 63 in 1750–69, 51.4 in 1770–89, but 41.3 by 1790–1809, a trend that was to continue throughout the nineteenth century, even though influenced by social class and circumstances. Of course, once the population had grown, an epidemic or harvest failure was far more serious, as in the Irish potato famine of the nineteenth century.

As well as the rising birth rate, a reduced death rate contributed substantially to the population growth and by the 1780s it was clearly falling. Better nutrition by the end of the eighteenth century must have played an important part and the bad harvests of 1793–5 and 1798–1801 affected the death rates less than those of earlier decades. Individual and community longevity was frequently noted in the press; thus in Derbyshire in 1797:

> In the small parish of Tibshelf ... which does not contain one hundred houses, there are now living betwixt 70 and 80 persons who are more than 60 years old, amongst whom there are 4 nearly 100 each, 18 betwixt 80 and 90 – and 22 above 70; a circumstance which perhaps cannot be equall'd in this kingdom.

Certainly the eighteenth century saw standards of living, with nutrition a vital part, improve for the mass of the English population. Labourers' wages were higher, a factor Adam Smith thought very important in population growth, improved agriculture meant that there was a greater, more varied overall food output in both crops and livestock, while better road and water transport by the later eighteenth century transformed distribution and meant that local famines could be averted. Eden's and Davies's enquiries in the late 1790s, however, suggest that nutrition per head among the very poor had not improved in step with the better distribution of supplies, from which the more prosperous benefited. Industrialisation undoubtedly created new consumer tastes, even among workers, and Malthus noted an increased demand for 'comfort and conveniences' in the population at large. Part of the growth in labourers' wages must have been due to their larger families, for even young children could earn and contribute to the family income, as David Davies illustrated in his survey of 1795 and writers such as William Hutton recalled. Of course, their earnings may not have equalled the additional expense of keeping the children until they could work, but Malthus was convinced that the prospect of parish relief and children's wages encouraged earlier marriages and larger families, a view echoed by the 1834 Poor Law Commissioners.

That the total population of England was increasing by the later eighteenth century and into the nineteenth, whether by more live births or greater longevity, was not disputed. Contemporaries' comments that paupers deliberately had large families so that they could profit from the Poor Law of course presupposed that conception was in some way a matter of choice. Even in ancient times such natural substances as lemon juice and vinegar were used to change the acidity of the vagina, or acacia, which ferments into lactic acid, as a spermicide. The essential difference between male and female contraception was that whereas men wished to avoid sexual disease, women wished to avoid pregnancy. In ancient times Chinese women took small doses of mercury as an abortifacient, while a cut lemon served as a cervical cap and pebbles were used as an inter-uterine device. However, female contraception, such as douches and soaked sponges, was available only to the affluent in eighteenth-century England, although Jeremy Bentham recommended the sponge as a contraceptive to reduce the poor rates in 1797. Folk and herbal abortifacients were widely known, including ergot, black hellebore, pennyroyal, garden rue and white saxifrage, which were also noted in respectable herbals to restore menstruation. Gin's popularity in abortions was due to its flavouring of juniper berries, a recognised abortificient, rather than the effect of the alcohol. In the nineteenth century hot baths and violent exercise, including cycling, were thought to induce abortions and Lady Stanley of Alderley (1807–95) wrote to her husband that the tenth of her thirteen pregnancies had been successfully ended in 1847 by means of 'a hot bath, a tremendous walk and a great dose'. Contemporary newspapers were able, with wider literacy and readership, to advertise in carefully-couched terms products that were clearly abortifacients, usually claiming to restore irregular menstruation. However, the morality of limiting fertility, especially among married couples, was much debated and avoiding conception was seen as flouting God's wish.

Women's fertility was substantially changed as breast-feeding was less widely practised; affluent ladies rejected it as unfashionable and restricting to their social lives, while poorer women wished to return to work after lying in. The Revd David Davies noted that women were 'mere wet nurses for ten or twelve years after marriage, being always either with child, or having a child at the breast'. Such a large poor family was occasionally noted in the press:

> We hear from Nottingham, that on Friday, the 11th instant, Mrs. Melvin of Bulwell, in that County, was safely delivered of a daughter, which is the 30th. time of her being with child. It is very remarkable that this good woman is now in the 45th. year of her age, and notwithstanding her having borne so many children, 17 of whom are living, she enjoys a good share of health and spirits.

At the time this was written, the maternal mortality rate was twenty-five in every thousand live births. Lactation was a passive form of family limitation and when wet nurses were hired, the mothers themselves, not breast feeding, began menstruating and were again pregnant quite quickly. There was also a traditional and widespread belief that the nursing mother should not engage in sexual intercourse. Indeed, by the middle of the eighteenth century, medical literature encouraged breast feeding for an appreciably shorter period, reducing from twenty-one months in the seventeenth century to twelve in the eighteenth, although William Cadogan and George Armstrong voiced medical opinion against 'mercenary nurses'. The many repetitive pregnancies endured by some women must have adversely affected their general health, even if they were prosperous, and women wrote to each other of welcoming 'the French lady' (menstruation) and warned each other against repeated pregnancies. Thus the Duchess of Leinster (1731–1814) had twenty-two children in thirty-one years, born at intervals of only eleven to fifteen months, the last when she was forty-seven. Only twelve survived into adulthood; the Duchess died aged eighty-two. Apart from such evidence, there is little information about when women became menopausal and thus free from child-bearing, although females occasionally noted in their family correspondence. Married couples seem to have used *coitus interruptus* to limit their families, from which quacks prospered as they sold preparations such as 'Strengthening Tincture' to counteract the feared weakening after-effects in the male. Unqualified practitioners actually promoted fears of *coitus interruptus* and offered cures for the debility, consumption, loss of hearing and sight that it was rumoured to cause in men.

Male contraceptives, although only for the prosperous and essentially to prevent sexually-transmitted infections, were used in England from at least the seventeenth century. In 1986 ten condoms made from sheep intestines were discovered when excavating the latrines at Dudley Castle, held by royalists during the Civil War, where officers and their wives lived during the lengthy siege. These condoms can be dated to 1647, some sixty years before any other evidence. They are of standard size and thickness, suggesting that they were made in quantity by a professional manufacturing process. Until this discovery, the other earliest examples, dated from 1790–1810, were the two specimens in the British Museum, still in paper wrappers. As early as 1564 the Italian anatomist, Fallopius, published a text, *De Morbo Gallico*, suggesting a linen sheath as a precaution against syphilis, and Madame de Sévigné in 1671 referred to the sheath as 'armour against enjoyment and a spider web against danger'. In 1760 Casanova thought condoms would 'put the fair sex under shelter from all fear'. The word itself was apparently not used until 1705; its origins are obscure, although the French considered it an English invention, using the phrase 'la capote anglaise' (the English cape) while the British had long used the term 'French letters' and 'condom' was certainly used in Daniel Turner's treatise on *Syphilis* (1717). Condoms were also mentioned in 1716 by John Gay in his poem, *The Petticoat:*

> The New Machine a sure Defence shall prove,
> And guard the sex against the Harm of Love,

and in 1726 Lord Hervey wrote to Henry Fox that he was sending him 'a dozen preservatives from Claps and impediments to procreation'. Boswell was unfortunately over-confident in his 'armour complete' of 1763 in his many encounters with prostitutes (Chapter 8) and on one occasion he recorded:

> I picked up a fresh, agreeable young girl called Alice Gibbs. We went
> down a lane to a snug place, and I took out my armour, but she begged
> that I might not put it on, as the sport was much pleasanter without it,
> and as she was quite safe.

Fear of infection from prostitutes, clearly illustrated in Hogarth's *Marriage à la mode* (1745) and in novels such as *Roderick Random*, meant that condoms were on sale in London brothels, primarily for men using prostitutes rather than to limit family size, and this undoubtedly made condoms unacceptable for respectable people. From the mid-eighteenth century condoms were also available from the best-known London wholesaler, Mrs Philips, who advertised in 1776 that she had traded for thirty-five years and exported goods to France and America. Male contraception, however, continued to be only for the wealthier and educated, until the efforts of Francis Place in the 1790s to promote birth control to the masses. He issued three handbills in favour of limiting families, based in part on his own struggles of marrying at nineteen and having a young family to support on his earnings as a tailor, as he budgeted to pay 'a medical man in good practice'. Although his leaflets were distributed in the industrial north and in London, his efforts were of little avail. The medical profession generally objected to the use of condoms as allowing promiscuity free from the punishment of pregnancy.

The coming of Goodyear's vulcanisation process in the USA in 1843, copied in England a year later, made condoms far more durable by treating the rubber with sulphur and heat. This new type of crepe rubber condom was widely available by the 1870s, some packets patriotically decorated with colour portraits of Queen Victoria and Gladstone. As infant mortality declined and women no longer expected half or more of their children to die young, birth control gradually became socially and economically desirable. Charles Bradlaugh MP publicly advocated contraception as early as 1862 in his newly-founded *National Reformer*; he was later, with Annie Besant, tried for publishing obscene material. Family size began to decline noticeably from the 1860s, with an annual birth-rate of 36.3 per 1,000, falling to 33 in a thousand by 1914. The leading early manufacturer of condoms in Britain was E. Lambert and Sons of Dalston, later The London Rubber Company, founded in 1877. In this year too the Malthusian League was formed, promoting contraception but advocating sponges for females rather than condoms. In the 1930s the invention of liquid latex to replace crepe rubber and the coming of automation meant that male contraceptives were produced for a mass market, cheaply and easily bought, and in two world wars they were to have a significant role in government attempts to control the spread of venereal diseases (see Chapters 8 and 10).

Induced abortion was condoned in the eighteenth century if it took place before the child quickened (the moment when life was thought to be present) and until 1803 it was not a criminal offence until fourteen weeks after conception. However, Daniel Defoe was outspoken against abortion in his *Conjugal Lewdness* (1727) as, later in the century, were feminists such as Mary Wollstonecraft. For the very grandest patients, qualified medical practitioners seem to have been willing to carry out an abortion, although naturally in the greatest secrecy, and William Hunter was alleged to have done so. They would also deliver an illegitimate child secretly for a wealthy patient. However, as late as 1780 it was possible for an abortionist to advertise his services in the *Morning Post*:

> Any Lady whose situation may require a temporary retirement, may be accommodated agreeable to her wishes in the house of a gentleman of eminence in the profession, where honour and secrecy may be depended on, and where every vestige of pregnancy is obliterated; or any Lady who wishes to become pregnant may have the causes of sterility removed in the safest manner.

Infanticide, of course, remained a desperate strategy, usually for the unmarried female and, although a capital charge, the eighteenth-century legal attitude can be seen to have slowly softened towards such cases in the courts. Most eighteenth-century local newspapers contain a striking range of descriptions of babies' bodies being discovered in suspicious circumstances:

Last Thursday the Bodies of two new-born Children, supposed to be
Twins, were plow'd up in a Field near Warwick: They were wrapt in a
Piece of an old Blanket, and one seem'd to have been scorch'd with
Fire, the other had an Orifice under its Ear, suppos'd to have been made
with a Penknife. 'Tis thought they had not been long buried for one of
'em voided its Excrements after it was taken up … . The Children were
Male and Female.

However, infanticide cases were noticed only when the perpetrators had failed
and a body was discovered. Indictments were never very numerous; for example,
there were only sixty-one cases at the Old Bailey in the years 1730–74. Death
usually took place immediately after birth, partly because the mother feared the
delivery would be discovered but also because the child might then be thought
to be stillborn. The 1624 Act (21 Jas I, c. 27), which was not repealed until 1803,
declared that concealment of a birth was a crime, including a stillbirth. The only
means of telling whether an infant had been born alive was the hydrostatic test
to see if the lungs would inflate in water, but it was inconclusive and William
Hunter cast doubts on its reliability. He urged judges and juries to consider the
accused's state of mind, for labour could deprive women of:

All judgement and rational conduct. They are delivered by themselves,
wherever they happen to retire in their fright and confusion … being
quite exhausted they faint away, and become insensible of what is
passing; and when they recover a little strength, find the child, whether
stillborn or not, is completely lifeless.

In his *Dissertation on Infanticide* (1821) William Hutchinson MD defined a live
birth as one capable of surviving outside the uterus and in the nineteenth
century insanity as an infanticide defence became more successful in the courts.
The Infanticide Acts of 1922 and 1938, echoing recent advances in psychiatric
medicine, declared that any woman killing a child under the age of twelve
months would be charged with the lesser crime of manslaughter rather than
murder, based on a plea of temporary insanity.

Female servants were, however, always the group of mothers most likely to
attempt to hide a pregnancy and risk infanticide since they would be discharged
and left to claim poor relief once the pregnancy was discovered. The risks to the
respectable female servant from her employers and other servants were graphically described in *Pamela* (1740), while a Northampton servant in 1759, executed for infanticide, told how 'her master was present when she was delivered
and that immediately after the birth he took the child from her, stabbed it and
put it into the necessary house'. The heaviest sentence for murder was that the
prisoner should be anatomised after being executed and in Wiltshire in the years
1752–96, for example, half of the twelve dissections ordered were to be on those
guilty of infanticide:

> 23 August 1779: Seend. A female infant bastard, born to Katherine
> Hill, single woman: murdered and thrown into a well by the mother;
> Mary Smart, her mistress, and John Ring, the child's father and Mary's
> brother, were privy and accessory to the same. Ring is absconded, Mary
> in Fisherton Anger gaol, and Katherine in Devizes prison.

At Salisbury assizes in March 1780 Mary Smart was acquitted but Katherine Hill
was sentenced to be hanged, her body to be delivered to Alexander Forsyth, a
surgeon, to be dissected. However, she was pardoned a month later.

An alternative to infanticide was 'dropping' or abandoning an unwanted new-
born infant where, the mother hoped, it would be found and cared for. Church
porches, the market square or the doorstep of a wealthy house were favoured
places and Thomas Coram claimed that he was motivated to establish the
Foundling Hospital in 1741 by the numbers of abandoned children he had seen
as he walked the streets of London. The hospital itself, however, was condemned
by some contemporaries as encouraging illegitimacy by providing shelter for the
foundlings and giving a 'premium for immorality'. Undeniably, unwanted pregnancies remained a problem, dramatically illustrated when the Foundling
Hospital announced an open general admission policy for a brief period in 1759,
during which illegitimate children would be admitted, irrespective of their age
and health, usually two vital criteria for foundlings to be accepted in the hospital. The response was overwhelming.

Women had continued to rely on quack preparations and abortions after
becoming pregnant in the absence of any form of contraception, although it is
clear from their correspondence that they often dreaded repeated pregnancies,
fearful for their own health, for their motherless children if they were to die, as
well as economic pressures when they could not work and as more infants survived to be maintained. Class differences, however, were noticeable by the early
twentieth century, and Marie Stopes (1880–1958) was particularly concerned at
the problems of poor women, especially the high maternal and infant mortality
rates. Work on contraception for the masses had been pioneered in America by
Margaret Sanger, who coined the phrase 'family limitation'. Marie Stopes in fact
condemned all the forms of contraception widely used in England – celibacy,
extended breast feeding, coitus interruptus, douches, condoms and abortion – and
promoted the cervical cap. This device had actually been invented in the 1830s,
but required professional fitting and was available only at a clinic. She published
Married Love and Wise Parenthood (both in 1918), but it was not until the
coming of her Mothers' Clinic for Birth Control in 1921 that the cap and the
diaphragm were available, albeit only for married women. The progress of her
clinics was slow and by 1930 the sixteen clinics and two private practitioners had
seen only 21,000 patients. The medical profession was uncooperative and recommended more safe hospital births as a solution. In 1927 the Public Morals
Committee declared that general access to contraception resulted in a 'poorer
hereditary stock'. Most British medical schools did not include contraception as

a lecture topic until the 1950s and government support was negligible. Only the Protestant churches accepted the necessity of family planning, while the Catholic Church remained resolutely opposed to all forms of 'artificial' contraception, advocating the rhythm method, nicknamed 'Vatican roulette' for its uncertainties. Abortionists of the 'back street' and respectable variety continued to practise illegally; the procedure was legalised in 1967.

However, the British birth rate fell noticeably in the twentieth century, from 34.1 per thousand in 1870–2, to 24.5 in 1910–12 and 15.8 in 1930–2, the only change a post war 'baby boom' in 1947 rising to 20.5 per thousand, and family planning became medically and socially acceptable. Reliable contraception for women, initially only for those who were married, was not to come for several decades in England in the forms of pill, coil, loop and implant, while condoms have been continually on sale.

The obstetric case notes of Thomas W. Jones of Henley-in-Arden, 1793

Case	Patient	Residence	Date	Child	Comments	£ s d
18	Mrs Foxall	Lapworth	13 Jan	son	A remarkable quick good labor	10 6
19	Mrs Harris	The Turnpike	10 Feb	son	Natural labor the greatest quantity Lochial discharge which I ever knew which of course made her weak	10 6
20	Mrs Lane	Wilmcote	22 Feb	daur	natural labour nothing remarkable occurred	10 6
21	Mrs Joseph Price	Wilmcote	28 Feb	son	natural labor do	10 6
22	Mrs Cranmore	near Royal Oak	6 Mar	son	natural labor do	10 6
23	Jos Bishops wife	Wootton	7 Mar	son	natural labor do	10 6
24	Wm Wagstaffs wife	Henley	24 Apr	daur	natural labor do	10 6
25	Thos Meads wife	Lapworth St	9 May	son	natural labor do	10 6
26	Seth (?)oys wife	Wilmcote	10 May	daur	natural labor, great looseness	10 6
27	Mrs Jennings	Yarningale	17 May	son	natural labor nothing particular	10 6
28	John Joyces wife –		26 May	son	natural labor nothing particular	10 6
29	Thos Shakespeares wife	Henley		son & daur	Complex Labour pains had been strong upon the Patient for 26 hours at least, her labor was accomplished without much trouble and nothing particular occurred more than Natl Labr	10 6
30	Mrs Davis	near Liveridge Hill	22 June	son	natural labor nothing particular	10 6
31	Mrs Clarke	Rookery	7 July		Premature Labor having completed only 30 weeks of Gestation	10 6
32	Mrs Barret	Wilmcote	10 July	son	natural labor nothing particular occurred	– –

Case	Patient	Residence	Date	Child	Comments	£ s d
33	Joseph Hopkin	Pinley Geeen	25 July	daur	natural labor do do	10 6
34	Mrs Baaylis	Liveridge Hill	6 Aug	son	natural labor do do	10 6
35	Mrs Hartley	Henley	7 Aug	son	natural labor the Child Still Born having a very large Hydrocephalus with scarcely any Ossification of the Bones of the Cranium	– –
36	Mrs Kendal	Rookery	9 Aug	son	natural labor nothing particular	10 6
37	Mrs Brown	Lowsonford	11 Aug	son	Preternatural labor the Feet presenting accompanied with the Furniss She was soon & safely delivered and as good a time as any common labor	10 6
38	John Joiners wife	Henley	2 Sept	son	natural labor nothing particular	10 6
39	Mrs Rd Taylor	Preston Field	15 Sept	daur	natural labor do do	10 6
40	Mrs Grissel	Beaudesert	21 Oct	son	natural labor do do	10 6
41	Mrs Sharmon	Claverdon	28 Oct	son	Difficult Labor A case of arrest within the Pelvis owing to a small portion of deformity in the inferior Aperture delivered with the Crotchet the woman doing remarkably well	10 6

Warwickshire County Record Office, CR 3019

A handbill to promote contraception, 1823

TO THE
MARRIED OF BOTH SEXES
OF THE
WORKING PEOPLE

This paper is address to the reasonable and considerate among you, the most numerous and most useful class of society. It is not intended to produce vice and debauchery, but to destroy vice, and put an end to debauchery.

It is a great truth, often told and never denied, that when there are too many working people in any trade or manufacture, they are worse paid than they ought to be paid, and are compelled to work more hours than they ought to work. When the number of working people in any trade or manufacture, has for some years been too great, wages are reduced very low, and the working people become little better than slaves...

You know all these evils too well. And, what, you ask is the remedy? How are we to avoid these miseries?

The answer is short and plain: the means are easy. Do as other people do, to avoid having more children than they wish to have, and can easily maintain. What is done by other people is this. A piece of soft sponge is tied by a bobbin or penny ribbon, and inserted just before the sexual intercourse takes place, and is withdrawn again as soon as it has taken place. Many tie a piece of sponge to each end of the ribbon, and they take care not to use the sponge again until it has been washed. If the sponge be large enough, that is; as large as a green walnut, or a small apple, it will prevent conception, and thus, without diminishing the pleasures of married life, or doing the least injury to the health of the most delicate women, both the woman and her husband will be saved from all the miseries which having too many children produces.

Norman Himes, *A Medical History of Contraception*, 1936, pp. 216–17

MEDICAL CARE UNDER THE
OLD AND THE NEW POOR LAW

Wm Horneblow for and in Consideration of the Sum of Ten Pounds Ten
Shillings to be paid (by) the said Over Seers of the Poor Covenants and
Agrees to attend upon and to Administer Assistance Medicines &c to all such
Poor People within the said Parish of Brailes as are Chargeable to the
said Parishioners.

Warwickshire County Record Office DR 308/60

Although the great Elizabethan Poor Law Act of 1601 (43 Eliz. I, *c.* 2) specified
the categories of parishioners who could be helped under its terms, namely the
old and disabled ('impotent'), poor children and the able-bodied unemployed,
medical care as such was not mentioned. Later in the century, the 1662 Act of
Settlement (13 and 14 Car. II, *c.*12) was equally concerned with remedies for
poverty rather than with treating the sick. Under its terms, the parish officials
were to 'set the poor on work' by providing the raw materials for employment
and workhouses, making cash payments to pauper families to supplement their
income and also giving the needy essential goods, such as food, fuel, clothing and
furniture. In addition, paupers' rents could be paid by the parish and their children apprenticed. In many ways this was almost total welfare provision. From
1662 the parish might also 'farm' the poor, often considered an economy, by
paying a lump sum to anyone who would completely maintain the parish
paupers, profiting from their labour in exchange. Farming the poor, however,
seems to have been fairly uncommon before the eighteenth century and even
then chiefly a strategy for large urban parishes.

The essentials of the Old Poor Law were the same in town or country, for it
was parish-based, locally-administered and small-scale. The parish was the means
of raising annual income to spend on the poor, based entirely on property owned
or rented there. Thus settlement rights were rigorously defended by the ratepayers and non-parishioners swiftly ejected from a parish where they had no right as
claimants. The system was relatively non-bureaucratic. However, it relied on
ratepayers electing parish office as Overseers of the Poor, usually two a year, and
on a basic ability to keep account ledgers. These accounts were inspected each
year by the county magistrates and instances of fraud were rare. Disputes,

however, were very common and all eighteenth-century English Quarter Sessions accounts are filled with inter-parochial quarrels about settlement claims, bastardy suits and removal orders, just as a hundred years earlier cases involving religious beliefs and practices had dominated. As a poverty strategy this was effective for the small rural populations of Stuart and early Georgian England, where officials knew all their fellow parishioners and when social mobility was generally low. It had always been more impersonal and difficult to implement poor relief in the large towns of the period, simply because of the numbers of claimants and a more shifting population. By the middle years of the eighteenth century, however, with unprecedented population increase, harvest crises, epidemics, the growth of towns and a vigorous economy encouraging mobility of labour, all poor relief became harsher and more structured. Although the workhouse has become the notorious symbol of the Poor Law, in the years before 1834 they existed in only a minority of parishes, mostly large urban centres, providing only minimal medical care.

In these changing circumstances the Overseers of the Poor nevertheless provided medical care for their parishioners, some paupers needing assistance only in crisis, such as in illness, others chronically sick, disabled or dying. Clearly, buying food, fuel, clothes and bedding could be critical for patients, but medical Poor Law provisions covered every aspect of primary health care, as well as some institutional facilities. An important and relatively under-exploited source for popular medical care are the thousands of account ledgers kept by the Overseers of the Poor across England from the seventeenth century until 1834. Those for the seventeenth century are predictably rarer than the nineteenth century's, but they do survive to give a remarkable and vivid picture of society. In addition, they are one of the few sources for the history of basic medical attention. Their survival, however, varies, so that, for example, of Warwickshire's 215 parishes only thirteen (6 per cent) have seventeenth-century Overseers' accounts, of which the earliest begins in 1623, while its neighbouring county, Gloucestershire, has thirty-two sets of accounts (11.4 per cent) for the years 1637–99. On the other hand, in the period 1700–50, thirty-three sets of Warwickshire accounts begin (15 per cent) and thirty-two sets for Gloucestershire.

Suggestions that the parish surgeon-apothecary was unqualified or of lesser status than his contemporaries cannot be substantiated by examination of Overseers' accounts, which also show, however, that empirics, quacks, bonesetters and the like were all employed by the parish officials to attend the poor, just as they treated the rest of society. The parish surgeon was the same practitioner who also treated others in the community, albeit with medications and for fees according to the patient's ability to pay. The distribution of medical practitioners in eighteenth-century England was such that many rural parishes were attended by a man who lived in the adjacent market town, where two or three individuals might practise. These men provided medical attention, often domiciliary, and medications, as well as delivering babies, performing surgery and inoculating against smallpox. They also had an increasing number of bureaucratic tasks as the century progressed – certifying militia men, inspecting factory apprentices, carrying out post mortem examinations and attending inquests.

The cheapest and first medical attention to the pauper was invariably for the surgeon to supply medicines, sometimes for pennies only. Some of these were not identified, merely noted as 'Ingrediences for John Taylor 2s. 6d.' in 1735 or 'pd the Apothecary for stuff to dress a child with Itch 3d.' in 1741. No matter how small the cost, Overseers' ledgers are packed with such entries. Very occasionally, the surgeon's receipts also have survived among parish papers, again meticulously noting even the smallest sums, such as those that made up a total bill of 10s. 8d. for one woman in the parish of Grendon:

(1769) 16 October dressing two blisters	1s 0d
Cerate	4d
a lotion	1s 3d
19 October box pills	1s 6d
ointment	1s 4d
3 November Cutting an Issue with all necessary applications	2s 0d
3 dose purging salts	9d
(1770) 16 January a lotion	1s 6d
purging pills	1s 0d

A substantial number of preparations were herb-based, often with folk origins, and such cures as aniseed water (at 6d. a pint), camomile, cowslip wine (for children ill with measles), elder ointment, linseed oil, liquorice powder and rhubarb (to produce 'violent purging') were all commonly prescribed by the surgeon-apothecary both for paupers and also for his more affluent patients. A wide range of unnamed palliative preparations was also used for the poor, for example, aperients (opening powders and deobstruent pills), blisters, electuaries, embrocations, emetics, salts, febrifuges (to reduce fevers at 2s. 6d. a pint), jalaps, liniments, ointments, salves, oils and bread poultices (to reduce swelling), all of which eased if they did not cure a patient's sufferings. Surgeons provided dressings and sometimes the parish would buy calico to make 'rollers' (long bandages). As well as purging, however, bleeding was an essential of eighteenth- and nineteenth-century medical practice, for all social classes, as losing blood was considered beneficial in most medical conditions. As well as venesection, entries for leeches were commonplace : 'bleeding Clamps child with leeches 1s.' (1792), '2 leeches on Ann King's temples by order of Mr Brown 1s. 8d.' (1806) although sometimes the task was carried out by an old village woman, rather than by the surgeon. Leeches cost 6d. each and for some patients, as in modern microsurgery, they were used to reduce swellings.

Parish surgeons used a vast array of named proprietary medicines, the most famous of which was undoubtedly Dr James's powder. Originally patented by Robert James, a Lichfield physician, in 1746 as an anti-malarial preparation, it was increasingly used as a general pain-killer; advertisements for the packets of powders at 2s. 6d. can be found in all eighteenth-century newspapers and indeed it was often sold by newspaper offices. Nearly as famous but cheaper at 1s. 3d. a bottle was Daffy's Cordial or Elixir, an opiate given for ague or for patients noted as 'very ill'. Godfrey's cordial was also widely used for sending fractious infants to sleep. In a similar cure-all category were Bateman's Drops, Dr Cole's ague draught, Costak's cordial, Freeman's drops, Gascoigne powder, Grant's drops (sometimes used for whooping cough), Dr Hooper's pills (for dysmenorrhoea), Ormskirk medicine (for rabid dog bites) and Spelsbury drops. Such medications were universally used in England, in some cases until early in the twentieth century, by all social classes.

The surgeon would make domiciliary visits to paupers to dress wounds and set fractures, to attend infectious diseases and deliver babies; he was in every sense a general practitioner. Many of the injuries recorded, especially at work, would be serious and life-threatening, even in the twentieth century, and the range treated by the parish surgeon was vast. Although many of the entries in the Overseers' accounts noted only that a pauper was 'lame' or had a 'bad' hand, others are striking in their details:

1781 expenses Carrying the Man down to Nuneaton that had his
Leg broke
Ale & Money to Nine Men 14s 11d
1789 Isaac Terry for board & nursing when his leg was broke 19s 5d
to journeys to D° 2s 0d
Mr Smart's bill for setting I. Terry's leg £4 6s 6d
1815 Mr Jones surg^n as per bill for journeys, medicines, cure
of lacerated wounds etc in Mary Pardoe when gored
with a cow £9 14s 9d

The number of surgical procedures recorded in eighteenth-century Overseers' accounts is inevitably small, but they were always relatively expensive for the ratepayers. Thus, in 1766 £2 2s. was paid to the surgeon for 'cutting Best's wife's back open', while in 1821 another parish paid £11 11s. 6d. to two surgeons for 'operation and Journeys and Medicines attending Elliott's wife as per their Bill'; the patient's husband was given 5s. in addition. An 'oppiration of the Stone & Gravel', however, incurred a charge of £1 16s. in 1826. Sometimes we know of an amputation only because the patient was later bought a wooden leg, generally for 5s. or 10s. Thus in 1826 £1 7s. was expended on '2 journeys to Birmingham with John Holmes's wife to have an artificial leg made and fitted'; she later had brandy by the surgeon's orders. However, some heroic surgery was undertaken, such as a mastectomy on a pauper for £8 8s. in the late eighteenth century.

As well as treating a wide range of common complaints, such as ague, consumption and rheumatism, the parish surgeon could also be called occasionally to the more unusual case. A fistula or ulcer, often persistent, always cost several guineas to treat, £5 5s. in 1791 or £6 6s. in 1822, for example. Another uncommon entry in Overseers' accounts were treatments for venereal infections, for which the parish authorities used qualified rather than quack practitioners:

1761 Dr Hollis for curing Sarah Burten of ye French pox	£3 3s 0d
1776 Dr Short for cureing John Monday as per Bill of the Veneral Disease	8s 6d
1818 Mr Gibbs for Hy Tompson with Aveneral disease	10s 6d

In 1781 the Brailes workhouse suffered an outbreak of venereal disease and the Overseers in this remote south Warwickshire parish paid £1 12s. 6d. for treating it. However, infected prostitutes were noted as commonplace in the London workhouses of the period and the old York workhouse had children lodged 'in the infectious wards with adults labouring under syphilis and gonorrhoea'.

A regular part of the parish surgeon's work was attending women in childbirth, although the majority of pauper women were delivered by the local midwife, usually unqualified. While every parish surgeon would undertake midwifery work, it is clear that certain practitioners, even by the mid-eighteenth century, were developing a local reputation as *accoucheurs*, to be summoned by the Overseers when a delivery was beyond the midwife's skill. When the surgeon was paid for 'laying' a pauper, his fee was 10s. 6d. or a guinea, depending how long the delivery took, whether he made more than one visit and if he were summoned at night or to a distant patient. These were, in fact, the fees charged for labourers' or artisans' wives, although middle class, gentry and aristocratic patients would invariably pay more, if only because they received several longer visits.

When, however, a normal delivery did not occur, the parish surgeon could be called to attend a stillbirth, a miscarriage or a woman who had survived an abortion. As well as herbal abortifacients, common in folk medicine, occasionally more drastic substances were used. Thus in 1795 a parish register noted the burial of a woman who 'killed herself by taking Mercury to destroy her Child'. In the whole area of forensic medicine the parish surgeon found his range of tasks expanding steadily throughout the eighteenth century. If only from the evidence in the press, as infanticide and child abuse became commoner or better-reported crimes in Georgian England, parish surgeons were increasingly called upon to participate at inquests and in coroners' courts. Their basic fee for attending an inquest was a guinea, but more if post mortem work were also done:

1766 Dr Gibbons attending the Inquest of Sarah Russell's child & at the Assize	£4 0s 0d
1771 Dr Harrold's bill for his attendance on the Coroner's Inquest & for his attendance at Warwick on Groves's trial [for murdering his wife]	£7 16s 0d
1779 Dr Wilmer attending Inquest on Mary Kimberley's child	£1 1s 0d
1780 pd the Surgeon for examining the body of Thos Savory drowned	£1 1s 0d

1796 Mr Welchman dissecting Wm Holloway	£1 11s 0d
1810 Dr Tookey attending the Inquisition on Joseph Adkins	£1 1s 0d
1810 Mr Soden bill opening & attending Inquest on Hannah Danels child	£3 3s 0d
1817 Dr Gibbs for attending & opening the body of Mary Palmer	£2 16s 0d
1833 Dr Jaggard attending 5 Inquests	£5 5s 0d

The expense and upheaval a pauper's suicide could cause a parish is clearly seen in one meticulously-noted tragedy from rural Warwickshire in 1773:

Mr Welchman coming to open Mary Buckingham having Poison'd herself	£1 1s 0d
Thos Kirby going to Warwick to fetch the Coroner, horse hire etc	5s 0d
Geo Watts coffin for Mary Buckingham	9s 0d
To myself ale that the Jury had	9s 4d
To the Minister & Clark burying	3s 0d
Anne Turner helping to lay out & attending when the coroner was there	7s 9d
Bread & ale for bearers carrying to Church etc	5s 0d

The Overseers spent a further 5s. 6d. moving the dead woman's goods, making a total of £3 5s. 7d., an unpredictable and unavoidable outlay from the parish's modest income for the year. At the time of her death there is no evidence that the family had ever been assisted by the parish, although her three children were later apprenticed by the Overseers.

In the early nineteenth century Henry Lilley Smith (see Chapter 5) noted how many labouring people suffered from ophthalmic problems and indeed payments for 'eye water' preparations are common in Overseers' accounts. However, ophthalmology seems to have been the earliest medical specialism to develop in the eighteenth century, for both prosperous and poor, although quacks continued to thrive. Parishioners with eye complaints were always potentially an expensive prospect for the Overseers, for, as treatment was invariably protracted, paupers would have to be maintained for several weeks if they were sent to a consultant some miles from their home. Thus in 1805 one parish noted paying 'Mr Boswell on John Smith's account taking him to Birmingham & the Doctor's bill for his eyes and maintenance at Birmingham 5 weeks £4 2s. 11d.', whereas Smith had cost only 3s. to keep for a week at home. Blind paupers, usually unable to support themselves, remained a long-term responsibility for any parish, as did psychiatric cases, and both groups were noticeable among permanent workhouse inhabitants, noted by George Crabbe as regular inmates.

How the parish paid the surgeon varied. Rural Overseers, in small parishes, even into the 1830s, were most likely to continue to pay him on a per capita basis for each patient attended, while in towns and large country parishes, even by the mid-eighteenth century, the annual contract was becoming common. Numbers were crucial to this choice, for it is clear that by about 1760 contracts were increasingly preferred as there were greater demands on the ratepayers and a more burdensome role for the Overseers. A contract meant that the parish would know in advance exactly what medical provision would cost for the coming year, so that, for example, an unexpected epidemic among the poor would not mean a large increase in the rates. For the surgeon, a contract assured his income for the year, paid in an annual sum, without the need to tender many small bills and wait for payment. Whether the paupers were worse attended under the contract than under the per capita system cannot unfortunately now be proved, since the medical contract has removed all the fine details of the accounts for the modern researcher. Overseers were, however, always anxious to control medical expenditure, and the parish officials of Stony Stratford in 1752 specifically ordered that their surgeon should 'not be paid any Bill for yᵉ Poor People if He Vissitts in any Sickness or Missfortune whithout yᵉ positive orders of one of yᵉ Overseers'.

All parish surgeons relied on non-pauper practice for their livelihood but the 1834 Poor Law Commissioners were sharply critical of the motives of contract surgeons, suggesting that such work was only a way to make a start in practice or undertaken simply to prevent a rival from doing the work. However, from the evidence of Overseers' accounts it is clear that well-reputed practitioners accepted contracts, especially in rural areas, qualified men who took substantial sums when indenturing apprentices and with prosperous fee-paying patients. We have no certain way of knowing if paupers were treated by the apprentices, although memoirs suggest that apprentices accompanied their masters on such work. Some practitioners undertook more than one parish contract in a year, thus in Warwickshire William Bindley of Nuneaton in 1775 agreed to a contract in both Bulkington for £6 6s. a year and in Nuneaton for £14 14s., two large industrial parishes; in Bulkington his contract represented only 1.5 per cent and in Nuneaton only 1.1 per cent of the year's expenditure on the poor. In the same county Bernard Geary Snow had contracts with four parishes of between six and ten guineas a year, as well as attending four other villages on a fee basis; he also carried out mass inoculation of the poor in one parish for £20. In some parishes the contract surgeon held office only on alternate years or by rota and by the early nineteenth century some urban contracts were arranged by competitive tender, as at Brighton in 1805 and Plymouth in 1821.

The actual terms of the contract for medical care varied in certain details, depending on the bargaining powers of both parties, a compromise between what the surgeon could negotiate and how little the parish would offer. The commonest format was for the surgeon simply to agree to look after the poor for a year for a stated sum of money, depending on the number of paupers, but some contracts specified that the practitioner was to provide midwifery, surgery and even pharmacy for the parish at no extra charge. Occasionally treatment of fractures and in epidemics was excluded from the annual fee. Before 1800 contracts for £5 a year in rural parishes were most commonly recorded, although as early as 1750 the fee was £30 a year in a city as large as Coventry. However, after 1800 a different picture emerges as a result of population growth and increased pauperism, alongside a hardening of attitudes to poverty and higher expectations of the medical profession itself, especially in terms of salaries. In one small county town, Warwick, for example, in the early 1820s the two parish surgeons each received £25 5s. for six months, which rose to £40 for the half-year by 1828. During this period the population of some six thousand hardly increased, but the level of pauperism and demands on the parish surgeons clearly did.

As well as qualified medical attention for the poor, there were also a variety of alternative practitioners the Overseers might employ. Their tasks covered a wide range and empirics treated conditions, often chronic, that were thought beneath the surgeon-apothecary's skills. They dressed wounds and let blood, they treated mastitis (breast abscesses) and skin complaints ('itch' and ringworm), always for very low charges; most had other employment, such as farriery. There were also eighteenth-century 'water doctors' or uroscopists, who would 'cast' a patient's urine sample and make a general diagnosis for sixpence or a shilling. A well-known midland uroscopist was Thomas Nash of Bromsgrove, who advertised his services widely in the regional press. The most significant unqualified practitioners, however, were the bonesetters, who would set a broken limb and manipulate a dislocated one. The bonesetter's skill was considered inherited rather than acquired and females practised alongside male members of their family; the legendary Mrs Sally Mapp of Epsom was herself a Wiltshire bonesetter's daughter. Two striking aspects of the bonesetters' work emerge from the Overseers' accounts – the low range of their fees and the long distances they would travel to visit paupers. The Matthews family of Epwell Mill, Oxfordshire, covered a twenty-mile radius and served over thirty Warwickshire parishes in the later eighteenth century. The family, including female members, continued to practise the art in the Midlands until the First World War. The Thomas family of Liverpool provides an interesting example of a bonesetting family that in the nineteenth century entered qualified medical practice, with Hugh Owen Thomas their best-known member, responsible for inventing Thomas's splint. The most commonly recorded entry of bonesetting was for broken legs, especially children's, with a fee of 5s. or 6s. in the late eighteenth century, increasing to 10s. 6d. by 1808 and to £1 by 1827. Plasters were used to immobilise a limb, dislocated joints were manipulated into place, cracked ribs were treated. Broken collar bones and shoulders cost more because difficult to immobilise, but manipulating or setting a hip or thigh was the most expensive of the bonesetter's procedures (£1 11s. for a hip, up to £2 12s. 6d. for a thigh). Even the female bonesetters travelled to treat paupers and in 1807 Susannah Matthews made a round trip of fifty miles, presumably by pillion, for a total charge of £1 18s. to set a broken shoulder.

For the most basic medical care, the parish paid local women, often themselves paupers, to attend the poor who needed home nursing, the bed-ridden and the dying, especially if they lived alone. In 1834 the Poor Law Commissioners noted payments for nursing to the patient's relatives as one of the abuses of the Old Poor Law, since paupers expected to be paid for the nursing attention the Commissioners considered was their familial duty, although such payments were recorded from at least the mid-eighteenth century as a means of giving small cash sums to otherwise poor parishioners. Such untrained women carried out the duties of an attendant or orderly rather than of a nurse; they were paid 2s. a week in the eighteenth century, which rose to 4s. by the nineteenth. They frequently took over general housekeeping tasks while acting as attendants. They would sometimes also lay out the former patient and prepare the corpse for burial, but this menial task was generally performed by old village women of even lower status than the nurses. Male paupers might be paid for sitting up at night with a sick man. The nursing of smallpox patients was for obvious reasons more dangerous and warranted a better rate of pay (see Chapter 8).

Midwives' services were in constant demand under the Old Poor Law and childbirth was a regular category of expenditure for the Overseers. The costs of childbirth normally covered the month of confinement, with cash sums of 15s. or £1 for the time the mother could not work or tend her family. Other charges were for food, drink, fuel, bedding and sometimes clothes for both mother and child, so that a single pauper birth could cost the parish as much as £5, as well as the future expenses of supporting a child and paying for an apprenticeship. For such practical reasons the Overseers were most unwilling for strangers to give birth within the parish, where a bastard child could claim future settlement rights, and moving on heavily-pregnant poor women was one of the widely-noted scandals of the Old Poor Law, although such Overseers' entries as 'midwife etc for tramping woman lying in 19s. 5d.' were commonplace in all areas. Some women were claimants only when giving birth. The midwives employed by the Overseers were almost entirely untrained, except by personal experience and observing deliveries. Their fee rose from 2s. 6d. to 5s. as the eighteenth century passed, often with their food and lodging costs as well, and by the nineteenth century some town parishes negotiated an annual contract fee with the midwife. Only the smallest community lacked a midwife who, unlike the parish nurse, was rarely a pauper herself.

As well as providing medical assistance, the parish also paid for artificial limbs, crutches and spectacles. Trusses were bought to ease hernias, a very common condition for the labourer and said to have afflicted between 10 and 14 per cent of the working population in 1786. The steel truss was widely sold at 10s. 6d. by the early nineteenth century, sometimes provided by the parish surgeon himself, but also by the growing number of specialist appliance makers to be found in large towns.

In addition to medical attention for the sick poor, the Overseers also regularly provided a wide variety of food, alcohol, household goods and fuel, as well as paying the costs of pauper christenings and burials, including the essential hospitality for such occasions. Sometimes the Overseers recorded only that they had provided 'table' or 'diet' in a pauper's illness, but on many occasions, if only to justify the expense to their fellow ratepayers, actual costs and quantities were entered. These details are one of the few sources, largely ignored in research terms, for the historian about the diet of paupers who were not in an institution. Dairy products, butter and cheese, were commonly provided, as was bread, for the sick poor. When meat was thought necessary for a patient, it was invariably mutton that was bought (3d. a pound in 1769, but 4½d. by 1799); beef was used only for making soups or broth. By 1832 one parish felt obliged to spend 5s. 'to Banham children being ill to buy some meat to strengthen them'. Sugar, at 9d. a pound in 1817, was a relative luxury and rarely provided by the parish, but malt, to brew beer, was regularly bought for the sick poor. The amounts and variety of alcohol purchased for sick paupers are perhaps surprising, but ale, brandy, gin, rum and wine were regularly entered in the Overseers' accounts. Ale was most commonly provided for nursing mothers to increase lactation, whereas brandy (at 1s. 6d. a pint in 1787, 2s. by 1807) was chiefly for those noted as very ill or near death. At a shilling a pint gin was also for the terminally ill and, like all alcohol except ale, had to be fetched to remote villages from the nearest market town. Although rum was almost exclusively for elderly male paupers, wine was provided for all categories of patients, including children, sometimes only for medicines to be taken in; occasionally wine would be bought because it was ordered by the parish surgeon. Buying food and alcohol for the sick remained a basic expense throughout the whole period of the Old Poor Law:

1815 for Thomas Barnicle	
bread	1s 7½d
bread, sugar and rushlights	1s 9½d
3½ lb mutton	1s 10½d
bread cheese & vinegar	1s 4d
ale & small beer	4s 8d

When pauper babies were baptised or any poor parishioner died, the Overseers paid for simple hospitality for the occasion, a christening or a funeral, usually ale, bread and cheese for the participants, costing a few shillings. Burial charges for a pauper could certainly mount up, as for John Freeman in 1757, who had a quart of raisin wine 1s., meat 1s. 6d., bread 3s. 6d., bread, ale and cheese at the funeral 4s. 6d., a shroud 4s. and a coffin 8s., a total of £1 2s. 6d., as well as nursing and coal. Such expenses, although not medical fees, were an important part of providing for sick paupers under the Old Poor Law.

Although the parish medical provisions were limited by the poor rate and the local surgeon's skill, from the mid-eighteenth century it is clear that numbers of parishes were becoming institutional subscribers to the new county infirmaries that were being founded (see Chapter 5) and thus able to have access to a wider range of treatments than the local surgeon-apothecary could provide and also to the skills of consultants, even if only one or two in-patients a year could be sent to hospital from a parish. By 1834 all English counties had at least one infirmary and many had a number of dispensaries to which Overseers could subscribe and where their paupers could be treated, thus considerably widening the medical attention that even the poorest might receive.

There was, in fact, no area of medical or welfare provision that the Old Poor Law authorities did not undertake; as in a modern welfare state they provided services from the cradle to the grave, albeit for only the technically poor in the parish, a category that most wished to avoid at all costs. Medical attention was from the qualified surgeon-apothecary, with the particular skills of the bonesetter or midwife in addition. The basic medicines were those provided for all patients except the most affluent and, although any practitioners would have spent longer with a prosperous patient than with a pauper, the same man treated both the lady of the manor and the parish poor. As can be seen from surviving practitioners' case books, the difference in status is firmly reflected in the fees paid.

Although there was a well-established medical service through the Overseers of the Poor, there were demands for change from the early nineteenth century, almost entirely based on the escalating costs of providing for the poor. When the Old Poor Law finally died, what replaced it was never to provide for the poorest people the comprehensive welfare service that had existed in England for nearly two hundred and fifty years. The welfare state was still more than a century away.

The New Poor Law

Although the Elizabethan Poor Law had functioned across the whole country for nearly two hundred and fifty years, by the 1830s there was very considerable disquiet about its administration, some widely-practised frauds and, above all, its vastly increased costs to the ratepayers. Not only were the prosperous dissatisfied with its operation, but the recipients of relief also felt they were harshly and unfairly used in many parishes when denied assistance from a source they had come to regard as their right, a view shared by some country gentry and clergy. Local variations were considerable, so that while paupers in small rural parishes were still treated in a traditional, fairly personal fashion by their Overseers, claimants in large urban areas increasingly suffered as their numbers swelled and the poor rate could not meet demands on it. In these urban parishes the wealthy ratepayers were few and often recently rich, certainly not with the traditional paternalistic view of their responsibility for the poor that was a factor in rural areas with old-style landowners.

Undoubtedly too the political situation caused many to fear. The Swing Riots provided a background of terror for English agriculture in the 1830s and this was to be matched by a similar outbreak of industrial unrest, as at Beck's Mill in Coventry in 1831, for example, although historians have shown relatively little interest in these town disturbances. Pressure for the franchise, Corn Law legislation and the unquiet situation in Europe added to the widespread climate of fear in England. The cholera epidemic of 1831 (see Chapter 8) highlighted critical social, medical and welfare problems linked to the whole question of the poor. The greatly increased population of England exacerbated all these difficulties.

Relief was seen as inadequate and yet expenditure on the poor was 'scandalous'. The Royal Commission of 1832 was the result.

The Commission of nine, with the Bishop of London as chairman, sent out Assistant Commissioners to some 3,000 of the 15,000 parishes in every county in England and Wales during the autumn of 1832. Apart from annual returns of expenditure on the poor, there had never before been a survey of poverty on this scale, for even Sir F. M. Eden reported on only a selection of parishes in the 1790s. The twenty-six investigators included Edwin Chadwick, the youngest at thirty-two, and they sought answers to sixty-two specific questions, with replies returned swiftly by the end of the year. The report became known for the notorious phrase 'less eligibility', defined as circumstances when the situation of the able-bodied person 'on the whole, shall not be made really or apparently so eligible as the situation of the independent labourer of the lowest class'. The Commissioners were convinced that 'every penny bestowed, that tends to render the condition of the pauper more eligible than that of the independent labourer, is a bounty on indolence and vice', a philosophy that immediately found widespread support among ratepayers. The changes recommended in the report comprised a hundred and fifty pages and were substantial, removing all claims to relief outside the workhouse except in apprenticeship and medical care. When Assistant Commissioner Charles Pelham Villiers, MP (1802–98) visited the four counties of North Devon, Gloucestershire, Warwickshire and Worcestershire he noted serious abuses in the Poor Law and some financial irregularities. He was particularly interested in existing workhouses, their diets, costs and inmates, including the special sick and low diets at Birmingham, with 'wine etc. as prescribed by the surgeons'. He was convinced that paupers in the workhouse were in a better condition than those outside its walls, but he also saw relief as a pauper's right, and that it was a violation of a poor man's rights to withhold it. Perhaps predictably, the self-supporting dispensaries founded by Henry Lilley Smith in the Midlands especially earned his favourable comments (see Chapter 5).

Bastardy was clearly a preoccupation of both ratepayers and the Poor Law Commission, with a 'prevalent belief that bastardy is extending under the influence of the law itself'. Thomas Jones, a surgeon-apothecary with an extensive obstetric practice in south Warwickshire, stated that 'it was not unusual for him, as an *accoucheur*, to deliver girls of 15 of bastard children', although he noted only one girl claiming to be fourteen and a half and another of sixteen among the twenty-one bastard births out of 422 he recorded in his case book of the 1790s. In an industrial parish with a population of 1,792 in 1831, Bulkington, in the north of the same county, the incumbent thought nineteen of every twenty brides were pregnant. However, the parish registers of marriage and baptism for Bulkington indicate that, in the thirty-six weddings in the three years from 1830 to 1832, only six brides were between three and six months pregnant. In the same registers in that period there were also surprisingly only two bastards baptised, although the Overseers' accounts show a high rate of illegitimate births and parish medical care for both mothers and babies. A similarly depraved picture of pauper morality was presented at neighbouring Nuneaton, with a population of 7,799, where:

> The solicitor to the parish, Mr Greenway, stated, that his house looked into the church-yard; that he was in the habit purposely of watching the persons resorting to the church for marriage, and that he could confidently say, that 17 out of every 20 of the female poor who went there to be married were far advanced in pregnancy.

Such sweeping generalisations from reputable witnesses were clearly very credible and welcome evidence to the Commission, supporting as they did a widely-held view of poor relief and paupers' behaviour, which would be amended if relief were restricted.

The costs of illness to a poor family were considerable, well beyond their means even if not regular paupers, and the 1836 Commissioners noted that 'in the matter of relief by medicine almost all rural labourers were paupers'. The answer to all the problems of poverty, including its escalating costs, was seen as the Union workhouse. Entry into the workhouse would be compulsory if relief were to be paid and outdoor relief, the mainstay of the Old Poor Law, was to be abolished. No longer would paupers receive cash, food, goods or rent in their own homes. The family would also be split up, with adult males and females in separate workhouse sections, including even elderly husbands and wives who had been long married. Young children were accommodated with their mothers. In only two aspects of relief under the New Poor Law was help available outside the workhouse – apprenticeship and medical attention.

Specific medical facilities in a workhouse are essentially a feature of the New Poor Law. The evidence for the early existence of workhouses has long been debated by historians, but the first ones were essentially poorhouses, providing shelter for those described as 'the impotent poor' in the terms of the 1601 Act. The Act had authorised 'convenient houses of dwelling' to lodge the old, the very young and the disabled, not as a means of providing employment. Troublesome parishioners were sent to the House of Correction. Larger communities certainly organised such poorhouses from a surprisingly early period, not necessarily requiring the inmates to work, and often the only evidence for these establishments is to be found in a county's Quarter Sessions proceedings when disputes occurred. There were a hundred established in the decade 1723–33. By the early eighteenth century, even before the 1723 Act in some cases, workhouses existed in towns such as Bristol (1696), Exeter (1701), Leicester (1714), Warwick (1717), Coventry (1724) and Leeds (1726). Evidence for medical provision is extremely sparse, but some workhouses, although intended to deter 'sturdy beggars', did add hospital facilities after their original foundation. Thus at Birmingham the workhouse was established in 1733 to hold six hundred inmates and built at a cost of some £1,200; from its early years a contract surgeon-apothecary and a midwife were regularly paid to attend the paupers. A purpose-built infirmary, costing £400, was added in 1766. Eden noted its considerable expenditure in the 1780s and 1790s. In 1789, for example, there were three surgeons, each paid £21 a year out of a medical total of £561 14s. 10d., which included £329 3s. spent on lunatics and £25 5s. on midwifery, as well as drugs and nursing charges.

When the House of Commons ordered a survey in 1776, there were 1,760 workhouses in the whole country holding 89,775 inmates, although a large county, such as Yorkshire, had thirty-five with 964 pauper residents. Eden had noted some workhouse infirmary facilities in the late 1790s, for example at Yarmouth, with two rooms for the sick, well-aired, and at Shrewsbury, with one room for fever cases and a separate infirmary with proper nurses. By 1815 there were 4,000 workhouses holding 100,000 paupers. Anxiety was acute by 1818 when 1,320 of every 10,000 inhabitants (one in eight) were paupers and, whatever calculations of poverty were adopted, pauperism was clearly seen to be increasing, especially in the form of outdoor relief, the most difficult form of assistance to predict and to control. As Colquhoun had commented in 1806, workhouses provided 'punishment without crime'. Larger workhouses founded in the early nineteenth century (under 22 Geo. IV, c. 38) seem little different from those established under the New Poor Law. The printed rules for one establishment specified the duties of the surgeon or apothecary, appointed by the visitor and guardians:

> [He shall] examine the paupers previous to their admission, shall visit the several persons in the house, at least once a week, or oftener if need be, and shall administer such medicines, and give such directions as to diet, as he thinks requisite; and shall make a report of the state of the poor in the house, and of the patients under his care, to the visitor and guardians, at the monthly meetings.

Institutions were perceived as the answer, even allowing for the considerable expense of erecting hundreds of workhouses across England in a short space of time, to reduce dependence on the Poor Law by providing facilities only the desperate would accept, in contrast to the lax regimes said to exist in the Old Poor Law 'pauper palaces'. As early as 1798 Malthus had favoured county workhouses 'for cases of extreme distress', not as 'comfortable asylums' but where 'the fare should be hard, and those that were able, obliged to work', while Bentham had proposed a scheme for five hundred workhouses, each for two thousand inmates, but with separate facilities for the sick and lunatic. In the New Poor Law scheme, thousands of traditional parishes were grouped into 643 New Poor Law unions, each with its own workhouse. The size of the county and its population obviously determined the number of unions, so that, for example, Gloucestershire had twenty, Warwickshire sixteen, Derbyshire nine, Berkshire and Oxfordshire only eight each. Even after a year of the New Poor Law, however, the Commissioners could report only fifteen English counties had formed Unions and elected Guardians, chiefly in East Anglia and the home counties. The 1834 Act recommended that the sick poor in the workhouse should be housed separately from the able-bodied with a less severe regimen; in the Commissioners' first report a year later there were model plans for union workhouses with infirmary facilities and nurses' accommodation (Figure 3.1).

The architect responsible for these model designs, extensively copied in the 1830s, was Sampson Kempthorne (1809–73) of Gloucester, who had Gilbert Scott as his assistant. Kempthorne built twelve new workhouses in nine counties in only three years, 1835–8.

Berkshire	Abingdon, Bradfield
Essex	Epping
Gloucestershire	Winchcombe, Thornbury
Hertfordshire	Bishop's Stortford
Oxfordshire	Banbury
Somerset	Bath
Surrey	Chertsey
Sussex	Ticehurst
Worcestershire	Upton-on-Severn, Martley

Kempthorne certainly gained these contracts because his father was friendly with one of the Poor Law Commissioners, but architectural competitions were often held when a new workhouse was proposed and these competitions forced the Guardians to improve the basic specifications of workhouses, under protests from the architects themselves at the low sums allocated for the new buildings. Some well-known men designed workhouses in the nineteenth century, including Lewis Vulliamy (1791–1871) and George Gilbert Scott (1811–78), who favoured the 'Elizabethan' architectural style and believed that a workhouse should be 'less a place of restraint than an asylum rendered necessary by misfortune'.

Several architects specialised in workhouse contracts, for example, in East Anglia W. J. Donthorne built eight and William Thorold seven, while the partnership of Scott and Moffatt erected over fifty workhouses in the 1830s and 1840s, favouring the classical style. The essential Kempthorne plans (cruciform or Y-design) provided specific accommodation for sick inmates on the first floor. His cruciform plan for two to four hundred paupers had twelve beds for women and twelve for men patients, while an alternative had twelve beds for lying-in, eleven for other female cases and twelve for males. There was also a nurse's room and a surgery on the plan. His standard Y-design, with three wings and three storeys, as at Abingdon, for five hundred inmates and costing £9,000, provided fourteen lying-in beds, as well as sixteen for women and the same number for men. At Chesterton Union the workhouse, with John Smith as its architect, was completed in 1838, cost £5,716 and was based on a Kempthorne plan; it is still a hospital. The Union workhouses were built either on the edge of a market town, as at Banbury and Hereford, or out in the countryside, as at Belper; they were sited some twenty miles apart, for it was thought reasonable that paupers should

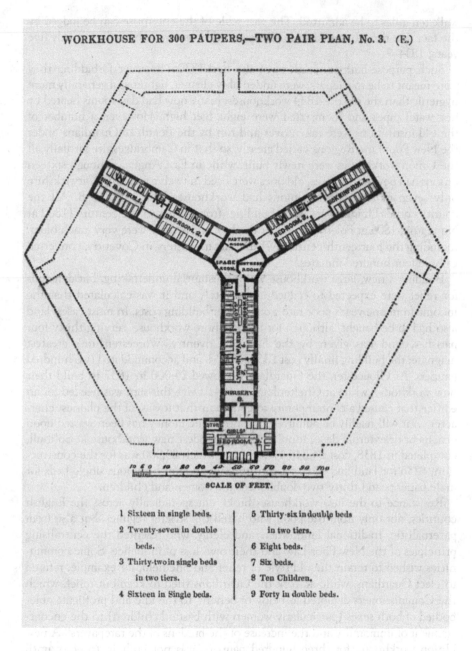

Figure 3.1 New Poor Law model workhouse plan from the *First Annual Report of the Poor Law Commissioners for England and Wales*, 1835.

walk ten miles to be admitted. The vast scale of the enterprise can be judged by the fact that three hundred and fifty new workhouses were built during only five years, 1834–9.

Such purpose-built institutions of the mid-1830s, however forbidding they were meant to be to paupers, were undeniably cleaner, lighter and generally more hygienic than the old pre-1834 workhouses; many now had day-rooms heated by hot water pipes and rooms that were eight feet high. However, a number of the old institutions were taken over and run by the Boards of Guardians under the New Poor Law. Regions varied greatly, so that in Cambridgeshire virtually all the Union workhouses were newly built, while in East Anglia, although sixteen unions had new workhouses, old ones were used in twelve areas. In Warwickshire only seven of the sixteen Unions had workhouses built in 1837–8. All the county's other Unions were using buildings from earlier in the century (1800 at Nuneaton, 1805 at Foleshill, 1818 at Rugby), while some were very much older, including the fourteenth-century Whitefriars monastery in Coventry, converted to hold four hundred inmates.

Building a new, large workhouse was a substantial undertaking, but demands for relief were expected to reduce immediately and it was calculated that the income from one year's poor rate would cover building costs. In most cases, land also had to be bought, although for the Pershore workhouse, serving thirty-four parishes, land was given by the Earl of Coventry, Worcestershire's greatest magnate; the building finally cost £3575 2s. 2d. and accommodated two hundred paupers. At Gloucester, the Guardians borrowed £5,000 in 1837 to build their new workhouse, while at Cheltenham in 1841 twice this sum was needed for an edifice that caused a contemporary to comment that it was 'of the plainest character ... it will readily be admitted that no public money has been wasted upon ornament or external decoration'. Even the modest new workhouse at Solihull, completed in 1838, cost £4,248 17s. 11d., of which £3,500 was for the construction, £236 for land and £316 for furniture, including thirty-four single beds for male patients and thirty-two double beds for women and children.

Resistance to the new workhouses broke out sporadically across the English counties, not only from the poor, who hated the stricter regimes, but also from paternalistic, traditional landowners and clergy, who resented the centralising principles of the New Poor Law and their own loss of influence. Some communities wished to retain the old style of relief and Sheffield, for example, refused to elect Guardians, while at York the Guardians tried to keep out-relief, which the Commissioners deplored as being of benefit 'to the idle and profligate able-bodied of both sexes (particularly women with bastard children) to the encouragement of immorality and the increase of the burdens of the ratepayers'. A new Union workhouse, for three hundred paupers, was not built in the city until 1847. Although there had been protests at separating males from females on admission at Eastbourne as early as the spring of 1835, the first reported attack on a New Poor Law workhouse was in 1836 at Heckingham, where a reward of £600 was offered to catch the culprits, while fires also broke out at such new buildings as Saffron Walden and Budbury. A new workhouse at Depward had guards, while police protected the one at Cressenhall. Sometimes the man actually responsible for building the workhouse was attacked, as at Macclesfield, where an architect's design for a building to hold 580 paupers, costing £5,000, was abandoned and the builder abused, forcing him to modify the old workhouse rather than build anew.

Provision of facilities for the sick varied greatly in union buildings and it was not until the 1860s in Norfolk, for example, that the rural unions began to provide separate infirmary buildings or wards for infectious patients. Anne Digby has shown that as late as 1896 only eight Norfolk unions had such separate facilities as part of the workhouse. Some cities were equally slow to provide special accommodation, with Coventry workhouse, for example, adding infectious diseases facilities only in 1871, although by 1888 the workhouse had its own infirmary with seven wards and 132 patients. The lowest level of provision for fever cases, a hut in the workhouse grounds, existed for this period at Solihull, in the same county. However, by the later nineteenth century, with an overall decline in able-bodied pauper inmates, more space became available for infirmary rooms within the workhouse.

In some workhouses infirmary facilities were long overdue and even as late as 1856, when Joseph Rogers was appointed as Medical Officer at the Strand Union workhouse, Cleveland Street, London, he found no separate hospital building for its 500 inhabitants, only 8 per cent of whom were assessed as 'well'. In 1866 he founded the Association for the Improvement of London Workhouse Infirmaries and in the same year *The Lancet's* views on the state of these infirmaries resulted in a considerable public outcry, supported by a timely campaign in *The Builder*. A new model for a separate workhouse infirmary was designed by Thomas Worthington at Chorlton in 1864–5 on the pavilion principle. This infirmary could admit 480 patients, each of whom had 1,350 cubic feet of air space, a generous allocation but slightly below the ideal figure of 1,500 cubic feet. Florence Nightingale praised the design as 'a model to the whole country'. Other workhouse infirmaries followed the Chorlton design, including St George's, Fulham Road, by Henry Saxon Snell, which held the largest number of patients, 808, in the metropolis.

The obvious need for sick facilities in union workhouses could, however, be partly met by subscribing to a local hospital or dispensary, a stratagem that had been quite widely used under the Old Poor Law to give a far wider range of medical attention to paupers than was ever possible within the parish, especially if in a remote rural area. However, some cases had to be treated in the workhouse that had been refused by the voluntary infirmaries, as one surgeon complained to his Board of Guardians in 1878 that 'cases of all descriptions, medical, surgical and even inebriates while in an intoxicated condition are sent into the Union infirmary for treatment'. He then listed the cases in this category he had recently been obliged to accept, including a servant with puerperal fever, another with acute syphilis, a woman said to be 'very exhausted' and a man with 'severe and extensive burns'.

Although there was no contemporary scientific understanding of satisfactory dietary levels for the sick, the diet within union workhouses was of almost obsessive interest to nineteenth-century commentators, particularly its financial cost. The 1834 Commissioners were especially eager to note what inmates ate and drank and in some areas quoted in detail the dietary provided for the sick. The workhouse food must have been extremely monotonous, but generally seems to have been adequate in quantity and it has been calculated that the weekly intake at the Easingwold workhouse was some 2,000 calories, nowadays considered adequate for a male manual worker. At Birmingham, C. P. Villiers reported the following ordinary diet, which he thought would attract the poor into an institution rather than deter them:

	Breakfast	Dinner	Supper
Sunday	rice milk	beef, vegetables, beer	broth with bread
Monday	milk porridge and bread	bread, cheese, beer	milk porridge and bread
Tuesday	as Monday	as Sunday	as Sunday
Wednesday	as Monday	pea-soup or Irish stew	as Monday
Thursday	as Sunday	as Sunday	as Sunday
Friday	as Monday	as Monday	as Monday
Saturday	as Monday	as Wednesday	as Monday

The 'Sick Diet' was noted as 'The same as the ordinary diet, only that mutton is allowed for dinner in the place of beef, and rice pudding instead of bread and cheese or soup'. Barley water as a beverage was allowed *ad libitum* and 'Wine, &c. as prescribed by the surgeons'.

Although buildings might be attacked, undoubtedly the most unpopular figure in the whole new system was the Relieving Officer, who was responsible for deciding which paupers should be given medical attention by the Medical Officer. No kind of qualification or experience was necessary to hold this badly-paid post, and at Ampthill the Relieving Officers were threatened by a local mob that 'we'll have the money out of your pockets and the blood out of your veins' if the old out-relief system were to cease. Near Royston in 1835 the Relieving Officer was threatened by a crowd containing numbers of women and one official was severely assaulted. The clash of views between Relieving Officers, workhouse surgeons and Boards of Guardians remained constant. With their Guardians' support, the Relieving Officers complained that Medical Officers ignored moral and economic factors in deciding whom to treat, the surgeons queried the Relieving Officer's competence to assess a pauper's medical needs and the poor themselves complained at the journeys to be made when they were ill, firstly to the Relieving Officer and then to the workhouse for medical attention, often travelling many miles. Eventually, yearly tickets were issued to the elderly and chronically sick to provide uninterrupted medical attention, without reapplying to the union officials. However, the national press in November 1844 was able to comment on

> the frightful mortality which appears to be the result of the administration of the New Poor Law. For the last month ... not a week has elapsed without the disclosure of some heartrending case, either of "death from destitution" out of the Workhouse or of gross "neglect of medical attendance" in it.
>
> The *News of the World*, 10 November 1844

Clearly the crucial figure in providing for the sick under the New Poor Law was the Medical Officer, who was required to be qualified, unlike parish surgeons before 1834, a fact much more easily ascertained after the 1858 *Medical Register* was published. The MO was appointed by the Guardians and the post was generally not well paid, but, as it provided a regular income in addition to fees from practice, posts usually attracted several applicants. The Guardians could clearly strike a harder bargain as a result of the increasing numbers of newly-qualified medical men seeking employment. In some areas the post would be advertised and Unions might invite local practitioners to tender, with Guardians naturally favouring the lowest estimate. MOs could be paid either an annual sum or on a per capita basis and the appointment usually created a post for an assistant in a practice, since workhouse demands on the MO were often considerable. The assistant was not required to be qualified and it was often found that a qualified man undertook the MO's duties and then his unqualified young assistant actually attended the paupers. One Hampshire practitioner, for example, in 1863, earned £140, a quarter of his total annual income of £576, from Poor Law work, and it has been suggested that two in five provincial practitioners undertook Poor Law work at some stage in their careers. Although many MOs may have seen Poor Law work as a chance to build up a practice, one of the 1834 Commissioners, E. C. Tufnell, considered that 'they are really and fully paid by the experience they acquire which brings them credit and private patients'. The growth of MOs may be seen in the near doubling of their numbers, from 2,680 in 1849 to 4,728 by 1906, at least partly in response to overall population growth in the later nineteenth century and more elderly paupers surviving to be attended. In the General Medical Order of 1842 it was decreed that the maximum district for a single MO should be 15,000 acres, but by 1861 there were 583 districts larger than this. A *Punch* cartoon of 1848 vividly illustrates contemporary views on the 'Splendid opening for a young medical man' that the Guardians could offer.

The levels of Poor Law medical salaries varied greatly even in one county, depending on the population and the MO's responsibilities. Thus at Coventry workhouse Charles Iliffe, the MO, began work in 1877, aged 36, at a salary of £60 a year; he held the post until 1911. However, at Solihull Thomas Lowe was appointed in 1839 at only £20 a year, providing all his own medicines and appliances; a substantial salary increase there did not occur until 1898, when Edward Page was to be paid £75, having accepted the post at £35 in 1869. It is not perhaps surprising that complaints, often of professional negligence, were made by the Guardians and the paupers themselves against these badly-paid and overworked practitioners, while the 1905 Poor Law Commission was severely critical of the workhouse hospital service, largely staffed on a part-time basis. Not all such men were of lowly status in their profession, so that Charles Iliffe also served as MOH for a Rural District and as Coroner for North Warwickshire for thirty years. A councillor and alderman, he lived in a large house on the city outskirts. Perhaps the most famous MO in the Victorian period, albeit for his non-medical activities, was the legendary cricketer, W. G. Grace, who served the Barton Regis Union, near Bristol, for twenty years until the Poor Law reforms of 1898. Some practitioners acted for very long periods in the office of Medical Officer, however, a fact noted on the tombstone of a Kenilworth surgeon, John Clarke, who died in 1894 at the age of seventy after forty-four years as MO for the district. The MOs formed themselves by the 1860s into the Poor Law Medical Officers' Association, while in London in 1866 the Association of Metropolitan Workhouse Medical Officers was established. The two groups merged two years later and were to be a strong influence on the growth of future medical services, gaining support from parliament, the BMA, the medical press and such famous contemporaries as Edwin Chadwick and Florence Nightingale. As a sign of the times, the journal, *The Hospital*, founded in 1886, included news about poor law infirmaries.

By the 1860s there was considerable pressure for reform. The medical profession was undeniably stronger after the 1858 Act and the *Medical Register* and, following the well-publicised deaths of two paupers in a London workhouse and general terror after the 1866–7 cholera outbreak, public opinion was in favour of change. The resulting Metropolitan Poor Law Amendment Act of 1867, later to affect the provinces, began the process of moving hospitals out of workhouses and medical need was to replace the philosophy of less eligibility for the sick poor. This was much slower to achieve in the provinces, and the 1905 Poor Law enquiry showed many hospitals still within workhouses. As late as 1899 there were 463 English authorities (32 per cent) paying their MOs only between £20 and £30 a year. Their workloads were large; for example, in 1865 it was calculated that in the metropolitan workhouses some 48 per cent of inmates were sick and in provincial institutions in 1869 the figure was nearly 30 per cent. When 128 unions were surveyed in 1907, the commonest illnesses were found to be primarily those of poor living, for in every thousand paupers forty-four had bronchitis or pneumonia, twenty had rheumatism or gout, sixteen had pulmonary tuberculosis and fourteen had heart disease.

The struggle to keep down spending on the poor continued throughout the nineteenth century and, although immediately after 1834 there was a remarkable reduction in the cost of relief, expenditure began to rise remorselessly by the next decade. Medical costs, however, were a very small and unchanging part of this expenditure, so that in 1840 out of a total of £4.5 million spent on the poor, medical services cost only £150,000 (3.3 per cent). By 1871 medical costs had doubled to £300,000 out of just under £8 million (3.7 per cent). The Guardians increasingly were used for implementing other health measures, such as compulsory vaccination in 1853, the Removal of Nuisances Act in 1855 and the Public Health Act in 1872.

Some considerable workhouse infirmaries were built in the provinces until the end of the nineteenth century, for example at Mansfield (1883), Lichfield and Dewsbury (1890), Sunderland (1893), Walsall and Whitehaven (1894) and by 1896 there were some 58,550 patients in Poor Law infirmaries or sick wards. In some parts of the country the Poor Law infirmary was in effect the general hospital for the area. Thus the Royal Commission on the Poor Laws (1905–9) referred to Camberwell Workhouse Infirmary as up to the standard of a first-class general hospital. It had 800 patients, 160 staff and five resident medical practitioners. The stigma of the workhouse remained, however, in baptism and burial, for although workhouse births were disguised in the parish register after 1904, workhouse deaths were still recorded as such until 1919; the word 'pauper' was not officially discouraged until 1931. Reform of Poor Law facilities in the early twentieth century was slow; a period of economic slump and international uncertainty, especially the coming of war in 1914, meant that money was not allocated to improve workhouse infirmaries or build new specialist institutions. There was moreover a widening gap between the better urban institutions and the traditional ones in rural areas, where mixed institutions still catered for the old, handicapped, unmarried mothers and vagrants, alongside the sick inmates. The stigma remained on entering a Poor Law infirmary and an admission order, signed by the Relieving Officer, was still necessary. Many of the 1830s buildings, ill-maintained, were still in use. It was not until the 1929 Local Government Bill began to dismantle the 1834 framework that true reforms were possible, paving the way finally to change the Poor Law medical provisions of a century before and turn over the hospital functions of the Poor Law to the major authorities. Under this Act about half of the 90,000 beds in England and Wales were appropriated by the Public Health Committees of local authorities to form the nucleus of their general hospitals and the Webbs considered the Act a 'sentence of death' on the Boards of Guardians. After the 1929 Act some Poor Law infirmaries changed their names in a conscious attempt to remove the pauper connection, thus Leeds Union Infirmary, built in 1874, became St James's Hospital, Camberwell became St Giles's, Salford became Hope Hospital and St George's, Fulham became St Stephen's. Many were to have key roles in the future National Health Service in 1948; in 1960 some 51 per cent of local authority accommodation was still in old workhouse buildings.

Medical expenses at Birmingham workhouse, 1743–4

		£ s d
28 January	Mr Audley's sallary	5 3 4
	laying 2 women in the House	3 0
1 April	Dr Nuttall's salary	4 3 4
27 May	Dr Audley's salary	4 3 4
22 July	Dr Birch salary	4 3 4
16 September	Dr Audley's salary	4 3 4
14 October	Mrs Pratt for laying Millward	1 6
18 November	Dr Birch salary	4 3 4
19 November	Wid. Groutage to send Edward Groutage to Guys Hospital	1 1 0
20 January	Dr Audley's salary	4 3 4
28 January	Wid Davis & children smallpox	2 6
24 February	Mr Green for a Wooden Leg for Greaves	10 6
23 March	Dr Birch salary	4 3 4
11 May	Wid Smith Bitt with a Mad Dog to go to Salt Water	13 0
6 July	John Taylor smallpox	1 0
27 July	Dr Birch salary	4 3 4
17 August	Sarah Watkins child smallpox	1 0
17 August	Mr Avery's bill Repairing and Whitewashing workhouse	6 6 0

Birmingham Archives, BRL, 380973

First annual report of the Poor Law Commissioners

Evidence of Mr. Thomas Brickwell, Surgeon of the Amersham Union

As you have been a medical officer under the contract framed on the system of payment per case, have the goodness to tell me whether you approve of the system of contract, and whether any beneficial results have followed its adoption?

I approve of the system, but the amount in the present contract is inadequate; I think I shall lose a guinea a week by it; in some of the parishes it is at present only one-third of what I have received in former years for the same time. But I approve of the system for these reasons: it is a self-acting check upon the relieving officer, in giving improper orders or withholding improper orders upon the applicant for medical relief, in making him feel that in receiving it he is a pauper, and causing the parish a specific charge for him, and upon the medical man by causing an inquiry into each case, so that none can escape attention, and by that means also secures proper attendance to the patient. Indeed the mode of contract forms a complete system of check and security, in cases of pauper medical relief, the want of which was so much felt under the old system.

First Annual Report of the Poor Law Commissioners for
England and Wales, 1835, pp. 263–4

4

MEDICAL CARE PROVIDED BY
FRIENDLY SOCIETIES

The Poor Man has his Club: he comes and spends
His hoarded pittance with his chosen friends;
Nor this alone, – a monthly dole he pays,
To be assisted when his health decays;

George Crabbe, *The Borough*, 1810

Thirty years ago it was asserted that the friendly societies of eighteenth-century England were an important 'unifying cultural experience' that 'crystallised an ethos of mutuality' amongst their members; William Hutton had described them two hundred years ago as 'this amiable body of men, marshalled to expel disease'. Modern research has concentrated on nineteenth-century societies, especially their links with the emerging trades unions, but largely ignored those of earlier centuries or their significant provisions for medical care. Eighteenth-century evidence is undeniably difficult to find, but as early as 1698 Daniel Defoe noted that friendly societies were 'very extensive' and, a century later, when Sir Frederic Morton Eden travelled round 38 English counties, he noted that a hundred individual communities out of the 165 places he surveyed had at least one friendly society, some with a hundred or more members in each. Eden was keenly interested in benefit societies as part of the contemporary struggle to control poverty and he regularly noted details of how they ran their feast days and funerals, as well as their sick pay and pension arrangements. All friendly societies had sets of printed rules and from these, in combination with the clubs' own cash books and miscellaneous papers, it is possible to see the vital role they played throughout the eighteenth and nineteenth centuries in providing health care and insurance for labourers and above – not paupers, but not so prosperous that they could afford entirely private medical care and fees. Indeed, those who had received parish relief were excluded from friendly society membership, although occasionally, as at Gnosall (founded by 1766), the Overseers would briefly take over a member's friendly society subscription to prevent its lapsing if his circumstances were temporarily difficult. In 1795 the Revd David Davies enthusiastically praised membership of friendly societies because they kept poorer parishioners 'free from the shame and misery of being burdensome to their parish, [having] it in their power to make for themselves a provision against sickness, accident, or old age'.

Distribution of friendly societies was uneven and differed in urban and rural parishes. Many societies limited their membership to a maximum (an odd number, to give the president a casting vote) and disappointed applicants often formed a rival club in the area. A geographically small catchment area for members was essential, since sick claimants were visited personally by club officials and the surgeon; in large communities a dozen or more clubs might exist with thousands of members. Thus by 1803 Birmingham had 7,253 friendly society members, Lichfield had 1,068, Worcester 1,189, and indeed the whole Black Country, with a substantial number of dangerous trades but relatively good wages, had the largest concentration of societies. Some clubs were definitely for only a single trade – shoemakers at Newcastle upon Tyne (founded in 1719), colliers at Hanham (1756), the Bristol carpenters (1768), the Carlisle cotton-stampers (1778), the London shipwrights (1793) or the Oldham spinners (1796). Non-manual occupations also formed clubs, for example, the Norwich musicians and the Covent Garden and Drury Lane actors. A minority of clubs were religious in origin, such as the Friendly Union of Cow Lane Chapel, Coventry (1778) or the society at St Margaret's, Durham for Anglicans only, while at both Ashford and Hereford there were societies exclusively for widows, the latter with 250 members in the 1790s.

The majority of clubs, however, were mixed as far as occupation was concerned, although a minority indicated their composition by title, of status (gentlemen, farmers, mechanics, tradesmen), of purpose (brotherly, amicable, provident, civil, philanthropic) or perhaps of political inclination (blue, loyal). All were single gender. Since they were essentially insurance organisations, criteria of age and state of health at joining were common to all clubs. Thus at Hereford men were to be between twenty and forty, with a certificate of their age, and at Ledbury the maximum age for membership was thirty-five. The Hanham colliers expected men to be 'healthful' and below forty, but was exceptional in not stating a minimum age at admission. Most men's clubs had age limits of between eighteen and forty, but a few societies (Dunchurch, Leamington Priors, Lichfield) allowed youths of only sixteen to join, although one of the most consistent complaints against the clubs was that they introduced the young to alcohol and public house culture. Some clubs, such as the Lancaster Loyal Union, with an age range of between eighteen and thirty-six, required extra contributions from members who were older. The oldest permitted age for membership appears to have been at Eccleshall, where men of fifty could belong. Most clubs expected members to live within a certain radius, not only to facilitate visiting sick claimants but for members to attend the compulsory social meetings.

Since a powerful motive for joining for poorer members was to avoid claiming parish relief, the club's benefit rates were critical and some societies held large sums of money. Eden noted in 1801 that total contributions in a year were over half a million pounds, 'an immense sum to be raised ... from those classes who subsist by manual labour'. He assessed each member's annual contribution to the box as 13s., but in the south of England contributions ranged from 1s. to 2s. a month. Although subscriptions varied, they were directly linked to the benefits paid. The majority of clubs required that 10d. at each monthly meeting be paid into the box to cover benefits. However, some clubs demanded more, so that at the Nag's Head, Chesterfield, members paid a shilling a month, at Lancaster Loyal Union 1s. 2d., while the Newcastle upon Tyne flaxdressers paid 1s. 3d. to the box, as well as 3d. for beer at their six-weekly meetings. At the other end of the scale, at Eccleshall only 4d. a month was paid and at Lichfield 6d. The usual amount for beer on club night was an extra 2d., making a shilling virtually the standard total sum spent. However, at the Bowling Green, Hereford, with the largest monthly beer allocation, 3d. was required. A clear relationship can be seen between subscriptions and benefits, an aspect of clubs that particularly interested Eden in the 1790s, for although regular contributions were the chief source of income, fines, sale of rules, donations, investments and occasional lottery wins all helped friendly societies. New members also paid an admission charge when joining of between a shilling and 10s. 6d.

Benefits remained the *raison d'être* for a friendly society, ensuring that the sick or disabled would not become pauperised and dependent on the Poor Law for assistance. These varied considerably, in weekly payments, in the length of the support period and the waiting time for benefit to begin. Some clubs specifically excluded certain medical conditions and social behaviour; there was often variety in the assistance given to members' dependants, for chronic illness and in old age. After Richard Price's actuarial theories were published in 1771, societies seem to have been more concerned with the factors affecting life expectancy and a number of later eighteenth-century clubs discriminated against particular occupations in their membership rules. All clubs required members to wait for one or two years after joining before benefits could be claimed and usually reduced the weekly sum after a specified period. Eden was critical of members having to wait for some time, as if on probation, before claiming. In some societies all calculations depended on the prosperity of the box, so that, for example, at Wolverley claimants had 6d. a week extra to the usual 7s. if the box held between £100 and £200; Eden noted similar arrangements at Caldbeck, Lancaster and Newcastle upon Tyne. However, benefits usually ranged from 3s. to the commonest sum of 6s. a week, while the most generous payments were of 7s. (Wolverley), 8s. (Chesterfield and Westbury) and 10s. 6d. at Hereford, where the highest subscriptions were levied. The lower rates were clearly not dissimilar to the weekly sums disbursed by the Overseers of the Poor to pauper parishioners (Chapter 3). Hutton noted that 'the charity of the club is also extended beyond the grave, and terminates with a present to the widow' and indeed fear of a pauper funeral and a destitute widow must have been a powerful factor in recruiting to men's clubs.

Benefits were normally lower after a specified period of illness, usually a year, by 2s. a week. Eden carefully compared Poor Law assistance to a Cumberland family, where the father, a labourer, received 6s. a week from his club for the first six weeks, reducing to 4s., but ensuring that he was not obliged to seek parish aid at a similar rate. A minority of clubs set out in their rules that members were 'not willing to be burthensome to the Parishes wherein [they] live' or did not wish to be 'troublesome to the Parishes they belong to', both statements made in the mid 1750s. Undoubtedly, fears of being destitute in old age were a considerable encouragement to membership of friendly societies, and Eden had noted that 4s. a week was the sum most commonly paid, although it could range from 3s. to 8s. for life. Some clubs had sliding scales for elderly members' payments, depending on their ages and how long they had been subscribing; thus at Wolverley members reaching sixty-five and not on the box were to have 3s. a week and 4s. a week at seventy, while at Leamington Priors 1s. a week was paid at sixty, 2s. at sixty-five and 3s. at seventy. Most clubs required members to have belonged for a minimum period before they were eligible for these particular benefits, for example, for fifteen years at Ledbury. In a well-run society, payments were arranged to balance subscriptions so that, in a society with modest contributions, as in the Becher Benefit Society for 1844, where 6d. a month was subscribed, benefits were 6s. a week in sickness, 2s. a month at the age of seventy and £5 on death. Since benefits depended on members' ages, a number of clubs demanded a certificate of age if this were doubtful. However, in most clubs, especially in those which limited their intake, presumably members of an age cohort from the locality knew each other from childhood and deception was difficult. Nevertheless, friendly society payments in old age were more than what the parish would pay, bore no stigma of pauperism and could reasonably be guaranteed, rather than being subject to the whims of the Poor Law officers.

Medical conditions for which benefits were paid were not usually specified in a club's rules, which invariably included only a general sentence of intent, for example, to:

> Glorify God, comfort and assist each other as Christian brethren, to
> provide for the sick and the lame, blind, prisoners, widows, orphans,
> aged infirm, and bury the dead ... to meet in a loving, peaceable, orderly
> and friendly manner; and by an equal contribution from each member
> to raise a fund for the support of each other, in the times of Sickness,
> Lameness, or Blindness.

Although societies did not specify medical complaints that were allowed for benefits, a minority listed conditions that were excluded, providing a rare picture of the health risks the eighteenth century saw in certain occupations, as well as in aspects of personal and sexual behaviour.

The trades that were widely acknowledged as hazardous, especially after the publication of Ramazzini's text book in 1713, were particularly related to the raw materials used by the worker, thus a minority of friendly societies either excluded certain workers or were formed exclusively for men in dangerous occupations.

Eden noted that chalk workers suffered from agues and at Lancaster members were not admitted if engaged in an unspecified 'pernicious business'. Those using lead in their work were widely regarded as most at risk and clubs excluding these men were noted by Eden at Stapleton, Nottingham and Kirkby Lonsdale. Since lead working was one of the main Derbyshire industries in the eighteenth century, it is not surprising that workers in the area formed their own sick clubs. Wirksworth had been the centre of lead mining since Roman times; in his travels Defoe described the local lead miner as 'lean as a skeleton, pale as a dead corpse …his flesh lank, and …something of the colour of lead itself', noting that he was also, presumably from brain damage, of a 'strange, turbulent, quarrelsome temper', all classic symptoms of lead poisoning. By 1795 the town had eight friendly societies with some 680 members from a population of about 2,800 (24.3 per cent); a third of the inhabitants worked in the lead mines and Eden noted eighteen miners' widows as needing parish aid. Other miners were also an excluded category and no 'pitman, collier, sinker or waterman' was allowed to join a Newcastle upon Tyne club early in the eighteenth century. Colliers also formed themselves into one-trade clubs, as at Hanham in 1756 or the Cumberland groups noted by Eden.

Others excluded from membership were almost universally unacceptable to clubs, either because of their occupations (bum bailiffs, merchants, publicans), or because they were serving in the armed forced as volunteers. Many clubs refused to accept members who already belonged to another friendly society. It has often been asserted that apprentices were excluded from membership, but this was in fact a very rare clause, although the Newcastle flaxdressers would not admit them. In practical terms apprentices, as unpaid workers, could not afford their club money and were frequently excluded because they were too young. At Leamington Priors both 'aliens' and Jews were excluded. The prosperous Bowling Green Club at Hereford permitted only householders to join, while the city's Coach and Horses Club rejected day labourers and servants, but both were unusual clauses.

Members' personal behaviour and responsibility for their own health, however, was universal in the club rules and benefits were not paid to a man hurt in a fight if he had been the aggressor, for a self-inflicted injury or to those suffering as a result of 'mobing' (being in a mob or a riot) playing football, using cudgels, jumping, wrestling or any 'needless past-time'. Men entering a club already having a venereal disease or becoming infected after joining were not entitled to benefit. The terminology for this exclusion varied, but 'French pox' was widely used, usually denying the subscriber for life. At Eccleshall one clause excluded any member who became ill by his 'irregular way of living or by any Notorious Vile Practice', which was unspecified. If there were any doubt whether a man had a venereal infection, at Hereford a physician was paid to examine him for symptoms. In one club, the Anglo Windmill, Coventry, the rules included the medical questions an intending member had to answer in person in the presence of the membership – his age, trade, whether ever subject to fits or other bodily infirmity and, if married, whether his wife were also healthy.

Those feigning illness were expelled from most societies and benefits were refused if members were found to be working, drinking or gambling while on the box. The Hanham colliers fined claimants for playing peck and toss or shake-hat on Sundays, exactly as depicted in Hogarth's third plate of *Industry and Idleness*. All gambling was forbidden on club nights, as were swearing, lying and profanity, while a number of clubs also forbade political comment. 'Disloyal reflections on the government' were banned at Ombersley, as was proposing a 'treasonable health' at Coventry. At Empingham Eden noted that friendly society members, who were in general poor, had made a collection to aid the Duke of York's army serving on the continent. This club also did not admit as a member anyone who was 'unfriendly to the present constitution of this country'. Most clubs forbade 'reflecting' on another member, especially by commenting that he was receiving club benefits, and some banned discussion of another man's religion. Some clubs expelled members accused of serious crimes, but later found innocent, while Ombersley did not permit 'abusive, obscene or filthy words' on club nights. Apparently unique, the Half Moon Club, established at Hereford in 1777, expelled members for adultery.

If members claimed benefit, they were visited at home by a club official and some societies had a rota for this task; usually societies did not expect an official to visit 'an infectious disorder whereof his life may be endangered' or, indeed, attend a smallpox victim's funeral. A minority of clubs paid a surgeon specifically for a diagnosis in a dubious medical disorder, while at Lichfield the practitioner was paid 1s. 6d. a head for each member in a five-mile radius and 2s. 6d. for each of two visits a week (maximum) for attending members who lived further afield. How surgeons and apothecaries were paid by the clubs is not always clear, largely because of the scarcity of surviving financial accounts. However, practitioners do not seem to have negotiated the kind of contracts increasingly found in larger parishes under the Old Poor Law, but to have been paid on a retainer basis. If a member feigned illness or tried to cheat the society, as at Hereford, a practitioner was to be paid a special fee out of the box to examine the claimant. As a further form of medical protection, a small minority of clubs became institutional subscribers to their county infirmaries, although they were far fewer than the parishes who contributed on the same basis. Thus in Oxfordshire the Bicester friendly society paid an annual two guineas to the Radcliffe Infirmary until 1788, but 98 other parishes in the county also subscribed, giving a wide access to hospital facilities. In Warwickshire by 1780 as well as three parishes there were also three Birmingham clubs subscribing to the town's new infirmary, whose admission registers indicate that patients were admitted when recommended by their societies, for example, a five-year-old boy with consumption sponsored by the steward of the Nag's Head club of workmen. The Worcester Infirmary had seventeen friendly societies as subscribers in the eighteenth century, some from beyond the county.

As well as the long-term sick, members who suffered accidents might in some societies receive special benefit rates; thus at Ledbury and Much Marcle extra relief was to be given if thought needful by a majority of the members for broken bones or 'extraordinary sickness'. At Epsom sums were specified and members were allowed £3 3s. for a broken leg or thigh, £2 2s. for a 'main arm bone' and £1 1s. for a fractured collarbone, rib or 'smallbone', in addition to regular benefit. Although chronic conditions must have been of great concern to the club officials, as to the Overseers of the Poor as a permanent drain on funds, at Ombersley no member was to be judged incurable until he had been on the box for six weeks at least.

Since friendly societies encouraged responsible, law-abiding personal behaviour, claims that sprang from dubious activities were not automatically paid and might be lengthily contested. Thus when one Derbyshire man had his hand shattered by 'the bursting of a gun' so that it had to be amputated, a long legal debate ensued about the nature of his sporting activities. His club rules clearly stated that any illness which resulted from 'unlawful exercise' should be denied benefit. This claimant left his house after midnight with a gun and was charged with poaching on private land, although he maintained that he thought it was common land and so was not trespassing. A barrister gave his opinion that the rules were intended to apply only to those acts which had a 'probable or immediate tendency to produce disease or bodily accidents' and thus carrying a loaded gun at midnight was permissible.

Recent work on women's friendly societies has concentrated on the nineteenth century, often with reference to Hardy's walking clubs, and there has been little research on the female clubs which flourished a hundred years earlier. All evidence suggests that eighteenth-century clubs were single-gender. However, the society founded by Boulton and Watt at their Soho factory near Birmingham began as a compulsory insurance organisation for all employees earning 2s. 6d. a week or more, with no exemptions. The distinction of being the first industrial friendly society appears to belong to Crowleys of Swalwell, an ironworks near Newcastle upon Tyne, in the early eighteenth century, but the Soho society must have been established by Boulton and Watt by 1770, soon after the factory was built in 1764. Although initially for men and women, a female society soon developed on its own and the main Soho club became a men's organisation. Some men's clubs were so opposed to the presence of women that their rules, as at Much Marcle and Ledbury, included a fine of 6d. for allowing a member's wife to enter on club nights.

The most urgent reasons for forming a women's society were twofold: first, that a man's club subscription covered only his own circumstances (injury, illness, death), usually also with a burial payment to his widow, and, second, that a pregnant married woman and an ill or unemployed spinster or widow could expect only parish help and became paupers when in need. Social events and companionship were, presumably, also attractive to women members. Eden was particularly interested in female clubs and noted northern ones that were thriving at Bury, Carlisle, Lancaster, Wigton and Workington. However, he also made an impassioned plea against the injustice of contemporary law that allowed a husband to seize his wife's club benefits, even though she had worked to pay the contributions, for 'where man is invested with arbitrary power, he will frequently abuse it'. In all, he noted thirty women's clubs and published the rules of two. In his sample labourer's budget he allowed 10s. 6d. a year for midwifery charges, twice the Overseers' fee to a midwife, based on a pregnancy every other year. Women's clubs ran on a smaller scale than men's, with lower subscriptions and benefits, fewer members and less ostentatious public events, but often with a distinguished and active patroness.

Surviving archive sources for women's clubs are extremely rare, but those that do exist show that female societies were at least as competent as the male clubs at managing their affairs, investing money and remaining solvent, although usually holding smaller funds. The Kenilworth women's club, founded in 1798, required only 1s. entrance money and 6d. a month subscription; members were paid 3s. 6d. a week benefit for a month and afterwards only 1s. 6d., with 10s. 6d. for a funeral and 7s. 6d. for lying in after giving birth, all very modest sums compared with male benefits. They had a much wider age range for membership than male clubs, essentially covering a woman's potential childbearing years from fifteen to fifty, but at Banbury the age limits were from sixteen to forty-six and at Chinley only fourteen to thirty-eight. Women's clubs do not seem to have excluded certain categories of members, as men's did, but Chinley would not accept any woman that 'hath any ailment or disorder upon her that may cause her to be expensive'. At the Kenilworth annual meeting tea and cakes were provided by the patronesses, whereas at Banbury members paid 2s. each for the feast day dinner and tea, held in the town hall. Like men on the box, women were not allowed to work (spin, knit, sew, wash, iron or outdoor work), but although ill, they were permitted to do housework, sweep, make beds and dress children. Women's societies demanded chaste behaviour; at Ashford and Chinley payments were withheld if illness were the result of intemperance or lewdness, at Kenilworth a bible and 5s. were given to a young member on her marriage, while all clubs, like the men's, levied fines for drunkenness at meeting nights. The justification for female clubs was succinctly set out in the preamble to the rules of the Kenilworth female society rules in 1798:

> It being usual for men to form themselves into clubs, for their support, under sickness and misfortunes, there seems to be no reason why women, who are exposed to equal if not greater sufferings, should not unite for the same good purpose, and from their own honest industry lay by a trifle for the hour of need.

Although there were various criticisms against men's clubs (dishonest use of funds, over-grand funerals, drunkenness), it was not until the very late eighteenth century that they were suspected of having political and trades union motives and therefore to be controlled. Rose's Act of 1793 required clubs to have their rules examined and to register at Quarter Sessions. They had always, however, been visible, public organisations, with annual sermons, processions, emblems and funerals, presumably to attract attention and aid recruitment. By the nineteenth century it was a mark of distinction for a club to boast of its age. In 1781 William Hutton noted that there were 'perhaps hundreds' of clubs in Birmingham established a century ago, while the publication in 1728 of a pamphlet advocating the regulation of societies suggests that they were numerous enough to create problems. It is, however, surprising to find societies established in relatively remote areas, as Eden considered that they were principally in populous districts. Colquhoun thought they had existed since c. 1700 and their numbers had increased since 1750.

Friendly societies always seem to have fascinated the contemporary press, when things went wrong (theft of funds) or for routine events (an annual sermon or dinner). Of particular interest, however, were instances of great longevity in their members, presumably a help to recruitment. Thus in 1812 the deaths of two very elderly members in different Warwickshire clubs were noted, a man of eighty-one at Stretton-on-Dunsmore, who had been a member since 1776, and another, blind for twenty-seven years, aged seventy-nine, who had received a total of £420 14s. 6d. (an average of 6s. a week) from the Southam friendly society in addition to £5 for his funeral. Clubs were, however, essentially organisations of interdependence and although they might own property and have gentry patrons, they were basically for mutual support, to protect members from reliance on the Poor Law in times of distress, sickness or death. It was as a shield against poverty, demanding individuals' effort and shared responsibility, that they were most praised by contemporaries and valued by those who joined. Refraining from claiming benefit was so highly regarded in some clubs that they gave an incentive to those who had never been on the box; at Much Marcle it was £5 after fifteen years.

Friendly societies functioned to a higher degree of literacy and numeracy than is often thought to have existed among eighteenth-century workers. They filled an important welfare role, making members both responsible for themselves and for other like-minded subscribers. Their role as providers of medical attention has been largely overlooked and certainly archival evidence is scarce. However, clubs always had a surgeon-apothecary, sometimes as a member, whom they could summon and certain societies negotiated a pro rata means of paying him – each member paid 1s. a year towards his salary at Stanton-by-Dale in 1785, for example, or 1s. 6d. in 1803 at Hopton, where the surgeon was to find medicines. At Hanley in 1788 his annual salary was £13, also including 'physic'. At Cannock the arrangements for employing the society's surgeon were set out in the club's printed rules of 1789:

> That on the club-night next before the feast, an able and experienced
> surgeon and apothecary shall be chosen by a majority of the members
> then present, to attend the sick and lame members of the society; that
> every member shall, yearly, on the feast day, pay to the said doctor, the

sum of *two shillings*: that the doctor shall not be obliged to visit the sick or lame members, who live at a greater distance than six miles from the club house. That if the doctor detects any member feigning himself sick or lame, in order to impose upon the society, he shall immediately give notice thereof to the stewards or clerk.

The problems of treating a society member who had left the club's area, often to find work, were considerable and archival evidence of medical attention, such as surgeons' certificates or letters, is scarcest of all. However, they must once have existed in considerable quantities and some survive to give an idea of how the system functioned. By the early nineteenth century some sets of rules printed a model surgeon's letter and certificate of illness, but typical ones seem to be those from J. M. Cater, a Staffordshire surgeon, in 1824 to the club officials in Derbyshire:

> Sir
> I am requested by Samuel Redfern a member of the friendly society meeting at the Anchor Inn Doveridge to inform you that he has been ill, ever since the beginning of September, he has left his situation 3 weeks ago and is now so infirm, as to be unable to take an active part in any sort of business, and trusts you will have the goodness to apprize the members of the club, that he is now under the necessity of declaring himself on the club box.
>
> Yours J. M. Cater
>
> 20 November 1824
> I do hereby certify that Samuel Redfern, member of the Doveridge friendly society is, on account of Rheumatism and other infirmities incapable of following his occupation and a proper object to receive the benefit of the club fund.
>
> J. M. Cater, surgeon, Abbots Bromley

The surgeon would for some patients even note a rate of benefit from the club, as in 1827 when W. A. Smith, MRCS (London) wrote that 'M. Kay a member of the Female Society at Barwick in Elmet has been for some time very lame and is not able to go about her business and requests the benefit of five shillings a week'.

Contemporaries undoubtedly saw friendly societies as a vital factor in reducing and even preventing poverty, illustrated in the *Abstract of Returns ...Relative to the Expence and Maintenance of the Poor in England* published in 1818, which devoted three columns to details about each county's friendly societies, citing, by place, the total numbers of club members for the years 1813–5. Two decades earlier Eden, in describing the state of the poor, had praised friendly societies and given them a prominent part in his survey, while George Crabbe's idealised picture of club membership was presumably based on his own experiences as both country surgeon and cleric in East Anglia and the Midlands. The fact that friendly societies were prepared to become institutional subscribers to infirmaries and dispensaries meant that their members had access to a far wider and more skilled range of treatments than could be provided by their own club surgeon. The membership comprised all social classes except paupers, with the support of honorary members and patrons, sometimes including medical practitioners.

The greatest change that came to medical services provided by the friendly societies was the development of the large affiliated northern orders in the nineteenth century, of whom the Oddfellows, Buffaloes and Foresters were the biggest, and the shift away from the local and independent clubs. At the peak of the self-help movement, in about 1900, at least half of all adult males in Britain belonged to these affiliated societies, although women were not recruited until the 1890s. Some required a minimum weekly wage among members (the Royal Standard Benefit Society demanded £1 4s.) and some excluded a particular occupation (Hearts of Oak Society would not accept miners), although only the Rechabites required teetotalism. The biggest orders, the Foresters and Oddfellows, however, had no such exclusions. Money remained a limiting factor in joining, for many clubs were charging members 4s. 6d. a week by the late nineteenth century, when a working man's wage was from 16s. to 20s. a week and, of course, employment had to be regular, not casual. The appeal of the societies was undoubtedly the level of benefits they paid, far ahead of poor law assistance and with no stigma attached; thus the Hearts of Oak Society paid 18s. a week and the Foresters 10s. or 12s. a week by the end of the nineteenth century. It has been estimated that 45 per cent of all working men had medical attention through the friendly societies by 1900. There were distinct regional differences in the pattern of friendly societies, emphasised in 1831 when a Select Committee of the House of Lords reported on the Poor Laws, for contemporaries clearly saw friendly society membership as a means of keeping down the poor rate. In their survey, the highest proportion of members (more than 10 per cent of the total population) was to be found in Lancashire, Staffordshire, Devon, Shropshire, Nottinghamshire, Warwickshire, Cornwall and Leicestershire, while in the areas round London, Berkshire, Buckinghamshire and Kent, there was thin support, as there was in the very remote, most traditional and non-industrial counties, such as Hereford and Westmorland.

The implications of this friendly society expansion for medical practice were considerable, especially for professional fees. Even for poorly paid friendly society posts, there were usually several medical applicants; at Worcester, for example, in 1871 there were thirty candidates for a post paying £170 a year and Lincoln Oddfellows in 1905 had twenty-two applicants for an annual salary of £240. Undoubtedly, the over-supply of practitioners enabled societies to negotiate ungenerous contract terms and after the 1840s more contracts included members' families to be attended for the fee. However, the contract fee often provided a substantial part of a practitioner's income, especially if newly qualified. Thus one Durham practitioner earned £126 11s. in the year 1846, of which £27 0s. 3d. (21.3 per cent) came from his friendly society work, while in the next year with a total of £167 6s., £57 4s. 9d. (34.2 per cent) was from this source. Moreover, friendly societies generally paid their practitioners promptly, unlike many private patients. However, the 1860s saw medical demands for higher fees, as more professional organisations were founded giving practitioners more authority. In addition, practitioners wished to exclude from the societies all those who could pay private fees for treatment, a growing number of the population as real wages increased substantially in the later nineteenth century. The dispute culminated in the 'Battle of the Clubs', described in *The Lancet* in 1896.

It is clear that the societies were considerably weakened by the coming of the National Insurance Act in 1911, which gave reasonably generous terms to practitioners, who received 7s. per capita a year for each patient, rising to 11s. in 1926. Other less obvious changes occurred early in the twentieth century, including complaints about the treatment provided by the societies' doctors, with a disputes procedure in place by 1899, as working class self-help gave way to a presumption of state welfare provisions. However, an earlier critic had told the Select Committee on Medical Relief in 1854 that 'the club patients do not get anything approaching the attendance which the paupers get from the medical officers of the unions'. A further advantage of the National Insurance scheme was that it gave the patient a choice of medical practitioner, an option not available to friendly society members, with no period of enforced waiting (three days in the Foresters) before seeing the practitioner.

Reflecting these changes, the societies' role in their community diminished, as they held fewer public processions and members participated less in meetings and feasts. In addition, there were considerable demands on their funds, firstly as death rates fell but longevity and sickness time increased, so that pensioners became a growing category requiring support. Secondly, reasons for claiming benefit had changed dramatically from the eighteenth century, when accidents outnumbered chronic conditions, to the twentieth, when the Registrar General's statistics show that heart disease (14.26 per cent) and tuberculosis (13.88) were the leading causes of death in 1908, with accidents accounting for less than 5 per cent. Also in the 1920s the societies' benefits had less purchasing power than formerly as prices rose, as did their own running costs, including medical incomes. The societies increasingly noticed in the twentieth century that claims for sickness benefit, real and spurious, grew as unemployment became worse. However, the coming of state old age pensions in 1909 and the National Insurance Act two years later were virtually the death knell of the friendly societies, whether independent or affiliated, and their arrangements, led by the 'ethos of mutuality', would not be equalled until the appearance of the welfare state in 1948.

Letter from Josiah Wedgwood to Robert Darwin about friendly societies, 1793

To Doctor Darwin, Shrewsbury. Etruria Feb. 7. 1793

Dear Doctor,

My son Jos has transmitted to me from London a letter of yours to him containing some queries respecting the influence of regulations among our workmen upon the parish rates. This, my Dear Sir, is a subject which it can do no good, and may do much harm, to bring publicly forward at all, for the most distant suggestion among workmen that they are investing their money to save the parish may do irreparable mischief. Some of the advantages and manufactures in a town and its vicinity are the great increase which they occasion in the rent of land and houses; the employing of the idle and keeping them out of mischief, and the increased consumption of all kinds of produce, an increase far more than sufficient to counterbalance any that can be supposed to take place in the poor rates. Though the regulations which workmen establish among themselves do certainly contribute much to lessen the parish rates by supporting in sickness and in old age those who would otherwise fall upon the parish, yet if the good effect of the Friendly Societies or Clubs was publicly urged as a motive for encouraging them, or as an instance of their utility, I fear it would be much more likely to retard than promote them. A few years ago a bill was brought into Parliament and printed for encouraging and promoting these societies. Some of the leading members did me the honour of consulting me on the subject, and desired me to give them my thoughts in writing upon the bill, which I did, and I shall not enclose you a copy so far as relates to this subject. The bill was rejected, and has not since passed in any form. Our Friendly Societies are the simplest things imaginable, a workman pays 2d. or 3d. per week, and receives 3 or 4 shillings per week when sick, and a less sum when superannuated. I heartily wish you success in your laudable endeavours to serve your town and neighbourhood.

E. Posner, 'Eighteenth-century health and
social service in the pottery industry of
North Staffordshire', *Medical History*, 18,
2 April 1974: 140

From the Rules and Orders of the Friendly Society of Tradesmen, Fowey, 1796

VII. That every member having made due payments for two years, and shall then, or at any time afterwards, (he still continuing a member of this society) happen to be sick, lame, or infirm, and not able to work for his livelihood, shall, during such infirmity (if confined to his bed-room) receive weekly out of the stock Seven Shillings; but in case he is not confined to his bed-room, and yet incapable of following his business, he shall then receive Three Shillings and Six-pence only, provided in both cases the growing income or stock will allow of the same. It is expected that the said sick member do apply to the surgeon of the society, or some other surgeon, who is to certify by letter or otherwise, the particulars of such sickness, at the next quarterly meeting, when he shall receive his pay.

XXI. That the surgeon be chosen by a majority, at a quarterly meeting; that he shall have an annual salary of fifteen pounds, to be paid out of the common stock; for which he is to take care of all sick members, except their disorder is, or came by the clap or French pox, or excessive drinking, cudgel-playing, wrestling, or fighting, (except in their own defence). He is not expected to attend any member more than six miles from the club-house. The surgeon not complying with the above rules, is subject to dismission.

Cornwall Record Office, DDX76/3

5

HOSPITALS AND DISPENSARIES

THE LINCOLN HOSPITAL was instituted in 1769. The governors at first hired a large house for that purpose; but have lately erected a plain, handsome and convenient building, consisting of four large and lofty wards ... in each of which are ten beds. At present, however, the fund of the charity allows only of the reception of twenty-four in, and thirty out-patients.

Samuel Foart Simmons, *The Medical Register for the Year 1783*, p. 86

The eighteenth century was undoubtedly the most remarkable period of hospital building in England, with twenty-nine new infirmaries erected in the provinces in the years 1736–97, five in London (1720–45) and a further five in Scotland (1729–98). The 1740s was the decade when most hospitals were founded, and political motives may well have played a part in this concentrated philanthropy, especially in the years following the 1745 Jacobite Rising or the later disorders of the food riots of 1766–7, when four infirmaries opened. There were, however, seven general hospitals in London by the 1780s, providing some two thousand beds, as many as in the rest of England. Unlike the workhouse building boom in the next century, hospitals were charities, funded by goodwill and generosity, run by volunteers, governors and trustees, and with honorary medical staff. Admission for patients was strictly limited to those deserving poor who had subscribers' recommendations, and these too were on a scale according to the size of subscriptions. In contrast, workhouses were open to all sick paupers. Patronage was clearly a crucial factor in the early success of an infirmary and, although a cleric was often an important figure in launching the project, as in the cathedral cities of Winchester, Exeter, Hereford and Worcester, the support of the leading local magnate was essential to attract and retain support. Thus Earl Spencer at Northampton, the Duke of Marlborough at Oxford, Lord Coventry at Worcester and the Earl of Radnor at Salisbury all served as Presidents of their local infirmaries, often for several decades and across generations, both subscribing and, more importantly, bringing contributions and support to the charity through their patronage. The Earl of Oxford, a prominent landowner in the county, gave the land on which the Hereford General Hospital was built in 1781. The northern hospitals, however, seem to have had a different pattern of charity, as at Sheffield, where £17,000 was collected before the foundation stone was laid in

1793, with leading local manufacturers heading their trustees. Only at Birmingham, where Dr John Ash was a founder, was the eighteenth-century medical profession involved in establishing an infirmary, although practitioners were usually important fund-raisers.

All hospitals used their local press initially to announce that an infirmary was being planned and subsequently to report on its annual progress and special events. Although these eighteenth-century county hospitals seemed to be local charities, five would take in patients from anywhere in the kingdom: Shrewsbury, Bath General, Stafford, Sheffield and the Radcliffe, Oxford. Some categories of patients were mentioned either for admission or exclusion. Thus Salisbury reserved five of its seventy-five beds for venereal patients, otherwise then admitted only at St Thomas's in London and later regularly an unacceptable category in hospitals, along with pregnant women, children under seven years, the infectious and the insane. Indeed John Guy, as a governor of St Thomas's, was so shocked at the excluded categories, that when he founded Guy's Hospital in 1724 for four hundred patients, both incurables and lunatics were admitted.

Sources of money were from individuals, by gifts, subscriptions and bequests, and from community efforts to raise cash, such as concerts, dinners, sermons and balls, as well as collecting boxes in local inns and the infirmary itself. All hospitals appear to have had financial support from well beyond their own county, with some wealthy aristocrats contributing generous sums to half a dozen infirmaries. On her death in 1766 the Countess of Monmouth left £500 each to Bath and Shrewsbury, as well as to eight London hospitals. For nearly three decades Viscount Dudley and Ward gave £10 10s. a year each to three midland hospitals, Worcester, Birmingham and Stafford, while Lord Coventry, president at Worcester Infirmary for half a century, gave £21 a year and left the hospital £200 at his death. However, benefactors' whims could be a factor in their generosity, so that, although Lady Elizabeth Hastings offered £1,000 towards a hospital in York, no progress was made and at her death in 1739 she bequeathed only £500 to the project. Gifts to a hospital in a benefactor's former home county, as with other charities, were commonplace. Some establishments were generously provided with land for the site free – as at Oxford and Hereford – or building materials – as at Bath, where Ralph Allen gave stone from his own quarries. A number of hospitals made use of a rented house in the town as temporary first accommodation, presumably before sufficient funds had been raised for a new edifice, but also to see how great the demand for admissions would be and what funds would be forthcoming. Northampton, Gloucester, Manchester, Lincoln, Hull, Worcester and Hereford all began in this way and raised money for permanent, purpose-built premises later.

Many eighteenth-century voluntary hospitals bear a striking external resemblance to the great country houses of the period. Several provincial hospitals were designed by well-reputed but not always first-rate architects, men who later flourished professionally in the area, with the infirmary as a good public advertisement of their work. Thus John Carr designed Lincoln in 1776–7 and Leeds in 1768–71, John Wood was responsible for Bath General (1738–42) and Salisbury (1767–71), while other infirmary architects included Stiff Leadbetter at Gloucester (1757–61) and Oxford (1759–67), as well as the Wyatts at Leicester (1768–70), Birmingham (1766) and Stafford (1769–72). A number of these infirmaries were justifiably described as 'elegant' and 'handsome' buildings. In their efforts to get the best value for the charity, trustees often considered competing designs from several architects; at Worcester, for example, in 1766 four men submitted plans for the new hospital, but those of Anthony Keck (1726–97) were chosen (Figure 5.1), one of his first commissions in what was to become a considerable architectural practice in the locality. At Worcester the total cost was £5,080 and Keck's fee, at £250, the usual 5 per cent. At Hereford in 1775 the trustees required 'on a healthful and airy situation … a plain edifice, recommended by convenience and simplicity … they wish to avoid … all useless and expensive ornament'; the maximum cost for the building, to accommodate eighty patients, was to be £6,000.

County and local involvement in the infirmary ensured that money would be carefully spent and the trustees themselves controlled finances, although there was also a treasurer, often a local banker, who balanced the accounts each year. Some of the hospitals, even as early as 1777, had substantial reserves of capital; Devon had £3,500 in the South Seas Company, Northampton had £3,800 in 3 per cent Consols, Gloucester had £18,000 and Newcastle upon Tyne over £5,000. A glance at any subscription list for the eighteenth century will reveal some very large donations and bequests; thus at Nottingham Henry Cavendish gave £6,337, while at Hereford there was one legacy of £5,000 and donations of

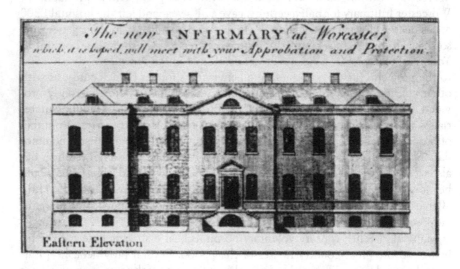

Figure 5.1 Elevation of the eastern front of Worcester Infirmary, 1767. (Privately owned.)

£500 (four), £200 (three), £150 (three) and £100 (eighteen) and various other sums, although £20 or guineas was particularly favoured (thirty-one). The nineteen donations of £100 or more comprised 75 per cent of the total capital there, while smaller sums of £10 or less made up only 4 per cent. However, at all institutions there were also donations of shillings. There were some supporters who were not wealthy but who could give modest gifts in kind to aid the infirmary and at Northampton in the first year, 1743, various local tradesmen gave such essentials as brushes, washing tubs, a frying pan and bellows alongside aristocratic guineas. Generally the local corporation contributed little more than a token sum to a new infirmary, for example, only £100 at Hereford, nothing at Leicester. Public support, however, in small sums of one or two guineas ensured a regular annual income and, perhaps even more importantly, an interest and involvement in the institution and its progress, emphasised each year as the annual reports were distributed, containing the subscribers' names and contributions alongside the statistics of patient numbers and expenses. The possibility of contact, however distant, with the governors and trustees must have encouraged some subscribers to participate. Most aristocratic hospital presidents seem to have been personally involved with the infirmary, not merely prestigious names on the annual reports, so that at Worcester, for example, the 6th Earl of Coventry personally chaired the majority of the annual meetings for over fifty years.

The design of the new infirmaries was perceived as an important factor to promote health, especially good ventilation, and for several hospitals the height of the wards, the number of beds in each and the window arrangements were emphasised when the institution was described. Thus Lincoln had four large, lofty wards, each with ten beds, all eight wards at Norwich were fifteen feet high and well ventilated, while at Liverpool thirteen beds were the maximum in any ward. The prison reformer, John Howard, approved the fact that Leeds Infirmary had ceilings 15 feet 8 inches high and that it was very clean, with uninfested beds. At the new Birmingham hospital, opened in 1779 with 120 beds, 'the wards are aired by means of three ventilators, and a circular aperture over each door'. At Manchester there was an awareness that death rates could be affected by poor ventilation, and in 1779 The Medical Register, having described the room layout in detail, noted that, in the rented house first used as a hospital there, of 403 patients admitted in three years, twenty-two had died, a death rate of 1:18, while in the new infirmary it was reduced to 1:24.5.

Being able to cite good statistics for curing or relieving patients was an important aspect of gaining subscriptions. Leeds Infirmary used the publicity value of their success rate in the local press in 1777, claiming that in the last year 926 patients were admitted, of whom 431 were discharged as cured (46.5 per cent) and 95 relieved; there were also 180 accident patients, of whom 145 were cured. To do this successfully, however, the hospital had to refuse to admit patients with certain medical conditions that were incurable and reject those who were unacceptable. Most of these categories in the nineteenth century were to be catered for in specialist institutions, such as children's, ophthalmic, venereal and fever hospitals. At Worcester in 1750 they were obliged to reject epileptics as in-patients, because their behaviour in the wards so distressed the other inmates. Every infirmary had a printed set of rules, frequently based on the earliest at Winchester, covering medical staff and subscribers as well as patients, but social control was strict and patients as 'objects of charity' were not allowed to drink, smoke, swear or leave the premises. Often cards, dice and other games were for-bidden, while many infirmaries required patients to attend prayers. Only those who could not pay for medical treatment were to be admitted, bringing adequate changes of clothing and letters of recommendation with them. Men and women were not to enter each others' wards and those discharged as successfully treated were to 'return thanks in their respective places of worship', giving a printed form to their minister to that effect. If the patient died, funeral charges were the responsibility of the subscriber and a deposit in advance was usually requested to defer the possible expenses of burial.

Patients were admitted once a week, for example, on Saturdays at 11 a.m. at Northampton, Worcester and Shrewsbury and on Fridays at 10 a.m. at Birmingham, although accidents could always be taken in at any time. If too many people arrived for the number of vacant beds, preference was given to those who had travelled furthest, presumably for those who lived closer to return a week later, and certainly in the years before 1800 patients might travel many miles to their nearest infirmary. There was constant contemporary concern at the running costs of hospitals and some governors published accumulated figures of how many patients had been treated over the years and at what cost. This was clearly an encouragement to ratepayers who would feel that they were, by their subscriptions, keeping down the expense of the poor rate and the costs of the workhouse, since the labouring poor, if cured by the infirmary, would speedily return to work and support their families without recourse to the parish. Basically, hospitals were seen as cost-effective. Such data were, of course, very easy to manipulate. Except at Stafford, where the two surgeons each received £30 a year, the medical staff and chaplains were not paid, while the apothecary, matron and nurses were poorly remunerated and suppliers to the hospital were expected to provide the cheapest goods for the charity. The annual reports make it clear, however, that treating more patients for less money was the trustees' aim.

Virtually all eighteenth-century provincial infirmaries were built in the county town and their coming must have had noticeable effects on the locality. In social terms, a hospital became the new focus of philanthropic efforts and subscribing was open to many of the middling sort who might not have participated in other ventures. A hospital was a large and noticeable structure, in the eighteenth century always sited fairly centrally in the town, that provided extra work and custom for the local craftsmen and traders. Its existence even encouraged new skilled men in the town, especially the surgeon's instrument maker, hitherto a London occupation, and in 1755, for example, Edward Cropper opened such a shop in Worcester, where his products would not have been needed earlier. The arrival of a hospital was always reflected in the county newspaper, where there were increased advertisements for medical books and more items of professional news, including appointments, marriages and deaths, as well as details about other hospitals. Thus, the *Worcester Journal* carried accounts of hospitals opening at Shrewsbury (1747) and Gloucester (1754), as well as regular reports of the city's own infirmary, including patient figures, dramatic operations, donations and annual sermons. It is striking how quickly a hospital might be created, so that at Nottingham, for example, in 1780 the new mayor allocated his feast money to the proposed infirmary, its foundation stone was laid in February 1781 and its doors were opened to patients nineteen months later, the building by John Simpson.

The presence of a hospital, not surprisingly, encouraged practitioners to settle in a town and the surgeons and physicians serving the infirmary were invariably the most senior men in the area, for such appointments were clearly seen as benefiting private practice. There were usually two to four honorary practitioners in each category, formally elected by the governors; they attended for one day a week and in emergencies, as well as for admitting patients. The day-to-day medical attention in the hospital, however, was provided by the house apothecary, a residential paid post. His salary seems to have related to the numbers of beds in the hospital, for at Worcester (with a maximum of sixty beds in the eighteenth century) the apothecary's salary grew from £20 in 1748, as paid at Northampton, to £30 in 1761, which it remained until the end of the century. He also usually had a modest annual gratuity of one or two guineas. However, in 1781 at Leeds, where there were sixty beds, the apothecary's post was advertised at £40 a year with the usual board and washing, while at Birmingham by 1818, although the salary was still only £40, there was also a £10 gratuity. The position of apothecary often attracted a number of applicants and at Derby in 1810, Henry Lilley Smith was one of the seven unsuccessful candidates for the new post, which was seen by some men as a career step before setting up in practice. In certain hospitals, as at Manchester, the apothecary was responsible for the general conduct of medical apprentices indentured to the physicians and surgeons. Governors' minutes and accounts suggest that when times were hard, savings were made on the drugs bill and the apothecary was clearly in a trusted position. His ledgers were always checked each year and his expenditure recorded in the annual reports, although the matron was usually responsible for the largest domestic part of the budget. Bigger infirmaries needed a paid administrative officer, while even small institutions had a hospital secretary who attended board meetings, prepared the annual reports and collected donations.

The changes in hospitals in the nineteenth century were in important areas; medical teaching and the whole profession expanded as never before, the acute sick came to outnumber the long-term chronic patients and specialist hospitals increasingly provided the newest kinds of treatment. At the same time a shift in influence occurred and the hospitals became more 'medicalised' as subscribers gradually lost their power to recommend patients and governors their day-to-day control of the institution itself. Indeed, the Royal Free Hospital was founded in

1828 as a protest against the power of governors' letters and selection of patients was increasingly based on doctors' recommendations. After the 1851 Poor Law Amendment Act guardians were allowed to subscribe and send paupers to hospitals and, as under the Old Poor Law, there is evidence in hospital admission registers that pauper patients were fairly regularly treated. At Birmingham, for example, in 1781 twenty-two parishes and eighteen friendly societies subscribed and at Oxford in 1799 there were 111 parishes and six clubs contributing, thus expanding the generally accepted range of those who might be admitted. Twenty-one parishes, not all in the county, subscribed to Worcester Infirmary and a dozen to the Shrewsbury Infirmary by 1780. Parish subscriptions varied considerably from one hospital to another, so that, for example, Norfolk Hospital excluded paupers because they had access to other medical services through their parish, while Exeter (founded in 1741) would not accept parish subscriptions until 1795 and the Radcliffe Infirmary refused workhouse inmates as patients for fear of infection; Shrewsbury Infirmary demanded a guinea deposit when admitting a pauper. However, Northampton Hospital actively sought parish subscriptions, with forty-eight contributing in the years 1765–74. Many of these eighteenth-century infirmaries were to grow considerably in the next hundred years:

Table 5.1   Numbers of patients at three provincial hospitals, 1892-1928

	Year	In-patients	Beds	Out-patients
Liverpool	1892	3,284		10,519
	1900	3,124	295	20,016
	1928	6,242	336	33,488
Northampton	1892	1,854		8,673
	1900	1,830	163	10,215
	1928	4,073	230	15,127
Shrewsbury	1892	1,163		6,405
	1900	1,126	120	4,318
	1928	1,652	130	4,131

The whole development of hospitals in the nineteenth and early twentieth centuries was inextricably linked to the workhouse infirmary (see Chapter 3), but an interesting small-scale innovation, the cottage hospital, was to make hospital facilities available to a different category of patients who were not eligible for, nor would wish to enter, the voluntary infirmary or workhouse hospital. The village of Cranleigh in Surrey has the distinction of having the first cottage hospital in England, converted in 1859 from a sixteenth-century hall, opened by a local practitioner, Albert Napper. His motives were both professional and social. He had seen in twenty years of rural practice that journeys to a distant large hospital were often impossible for the poorer labourers and their families wishing to visit them. He felt he could not give adequate medical attention to patients in 'the miserable abodes of the poor' and the coming of increased mechanisation meant that there were more serious farm and other accidents to be treated. In professional terms, Napper thought that the local gentry regarded highly only those practitioners who held hospital posts, an opportunity denied to most country doctors. Napper argued that the 'rustic labourer feels more at ease in lodgings similar to his own', but his idealised image of a cottage was closer to the Arts and Crafts Movement than the actual dwellings of the rural poor.

The concept of cottage hospitals was popular and Cranleigh's was followed by eight hospitals in five years, the earliest at Fowey (1860) and Bourton-on-the-Water (1861); 250 were established by 1880 and only Rutland and Huntingdon did not have them. There was considerable medical and popular interest in cottage hospitals, reflected in numerous publications in the 1860s. They were radically different from the great old voluntary hospitals in that patients paid a small sum for their treatment and time in hospital, often as little as 6d. a day, but were still admitted on the recommendation of an annual subscriber. They relied on the professional services of nearby GPs and, because cottage hospitals were so local, usually with fewer than twenty-five beds, providing a ratio of one bed for every thousand inhabitants in a rural area, local generosity was significant; Saffron Waldon's cottage hospital, for example, was built with a single bequest of £4,200. Some were founded by industrialists primarily for their own employees, as at Jarrow, where a hospital was built in 1870 by Charles Mack Palmer for his shipyard workforce. Cottage hospitals generated income of about £250 a year, only about a tenth of the total, from the 'deserving poor', but *The Builder* approvingly commented in 1877:

> The great feature to be recognised in the system is the requirement of a moderate payment by the patients, thus encouraging feelings of self-help and independence. We cannot resist the conviction that our great hospitals are great pauperising centres.

Most cottage hospitals admitted children and in the early twentieth century outpatients were increasingly treated, as were maternity cases. Some were built as war memorials after 1918, but generally they were superseded by larger general hospitals in towns and cities. The one major category of patients for whom there were still no provision, apart from the workhouse, were the chronic cases whose plight was ignored until tackled as a public health issue at the end of the nineteenth century.

Dispensaries

Although infirmary provisions grew steadily for a century after 1750, the out-patient figures alone suggest that there was a great unsatisfied demand for non-residential medical attention and, of course, out-patient numbers were limited because they also had to secure a letter of recommendation to be treated. The idea of a dispensary for the poor was first proposed as early as 1687, when the College of Physicians tried to establish one in London to restrict the growth of apothecary prescribing. By 1696 the London Dispensary for Sick Poor was established by the College, providing medicines at cost, with the physicians giving their services free. Predictably the apothecaries objected to such developments, and Sir Samuel Garth, himself a physician, had ridiculed their opposition in his burlesque poem, *The Dispensary* (1699). In the period 1701–4 the London Dispensary was said to have issued some 24,000 prescriptions a year. It lasted until 1725, but other dispensaries in the capital were not to follow for four decades. In 1769 George Armstrong set up a dispensary in Red Lion Square, London, for the relief of the infant poor, but it did not really mark the beginning of the dispensary movement. It was for only one category of patients, normally excluded by the voluntary infirmaries, and it was not until a year later, when J. C. Lettsom founded his General Dispensary at Aldersgate Street, that the true dispensary movement began in the capital.

Very early examples of dispensaries can be found in the provinces, at Bristol, where the Wesleyans founded one in 1747, and at Stroud, where a subscription dispensary was functioning by 1755, giving free medical treatment and served by a physician and two surgeons. It was said to accept five hundred patients a year, a substantial proportion of the population. In 1783 *The Medical Register* noted the existence of six provincial dispensaries, one of which, at Newbury, established in 1778, had recently closed. Their origins were varied. Two were the result of private initiative, for at Leicester Thomas Arnold opened a dispensary in 1776 after he resigned from the county hospital; patients there were required to pay a small sum for their medicines. At Bamburgh in Northumberland there was a general dispensary for the poor, open to all, supported by Lord Crewe's trustees; a blue flag flew when the surgeon was at the castle. There were also in-patient facilities and in 1782 nineteen sufferers were treated, although the infirmary was chiefly for sick and wounded seamen. In 1782 a total of 572 out-patients had attended.

At Newcastle upon Tyne a dispensary was founded in 1777, admitting two-thirds of its patients who were 'improper objects for the Infirmary'; 607 were treated in its first year, of whom 448 were said to be cured. A dispensary was founded at Liverpool a year later, based on the London dispensaries, and met with 'considerable encouragement', although initially it opened in a small rented house. So great was the demand from patients, that the governors bought land in the town centre and 'erected thereon a building, perhaps equal in elegance, size, and convenience, to any similar institution in the kingdom'. Apart from private voluntary contributions, the parish gave £105 a year to the dispensary. In its first four years, the dispensary had treated 37,580 patients; it was attended gratis by three physicians and three surgeons, as well as a resident apothecary.

In London, however, the growth in dispensaries was particularly striking in the nineteenth century and by 1861 there were thirty-nine dispensaries in the capital, as well as fourteen general and sixty-six special hospitals, all together giving a total of some 11,000 beds for the inhabitants. Such expansion was clearly linked to a larger population, the growth of the medical profession as a whole and the increased demand for teaching hospital facilities, both in the provinces and in London, where there were twelve hospitals with medical schools by 1858 (see Chapter 1). Many medical students in fact gained valuable experience by working in dispensaries as well as in hospitals.

Apart from general dispensaries, there were also a handful of specialist institutions catering for patients normally excluded from the voluntary infirmaries. Thus at Newcastle upon Tyne there was a Lying-In Hospital for poor married women and a Lying-In Charity for delivering them in their own homes, both founded in 1760, while at Bristol a dispensary, established in 1775, was expanded to treat poor inhabitants in their own homes, including pregnant women. Bristol Dispensary claimed to treat some four hundred poor a year, as well as 150 lying-in women, figures which rose by 1807 to two thousand and five hundred respectively.

However, it was not until well after 1800 that dispensaries can be seen scattered across the whole country, treating relatively large numbers of poor patients either free or for very modest sums. William Hutton emphasised that their role was:

> To supply the industrious of the labouring classes, who are not able to pay a surgeon for his services, with medical and surgical relief, for the payment of a trifling subscription. It also affords, by the contribution of the opulent and benevolent, relief to those who are unable to contribute any sum themselves.

Virtually all dispensaries were founded in populous towns, such as Bradford (1826–7), Birmingham (1828) and Newcastle upon Tyne (1839), rather than in the countryside. During the years 1808–32 there were also a total of nineteen specialist eye institutions founded in England, the majority by practitioners, including Exeter (1808), Bristol (1810 and 1812), Bath (1811), Taunton (1816), Hull (1822) and Birmingham (1828). If for no other reason, the work of Henry Lilley Smith and his self-supporting dispensary movement deserves reappraisal and greater recognition. He successfully brought dispensary facilities to a small Warwickshire market town, from where the concept spread to other communities in the Midlands and beyond.

Lilley Smith came from a Coventry trading family who had become minor landowners at Southam by the early nineteenth century. He was trained at Guy's Hospital, served briefly as an army surgeon and qualified as MRCS in 1810. In London he came to know John Cunningham Saunders, the founder of Moorfields Eye Hospital, whose work influenced Lilley Smith on his return to his family home in Warwickshire in 1810. In Southam Lilley Smith was employed as a parish surgeon, but deplored the Overseers' stratagem of farming out the sick poor for an annual contract sum, and in 1819 he published the first of many pamphlets on the medical care of the poor, *Observations on the Prevailing Practice of Supplying Medical Assistance to the Poor*. In his model parish dispensary there would be charitable contributions, members' subscriptions and parish subscriptions. The labourers would pay a weekly contribution and receive free medical attention, domiciliary visits and free medicines. The income would pay practitioners' fees, the dispenser's wage and the cost of drugs. There would be several practitioners serving the dispensary and patients could choose whom to consult. Midwifery was excluded at the beginning of his plans. He actively sought support for his ideas in the local and medical press, as well as sending copies of his publications to politicians. In 1823 he was able to open his 'self-supporting, parish and charitable dispensary' in Southam, followed by others in Leicester in 1826, Atherstone (1828), Coventry, Derby, Lymington and Northampton (all in 1831). Predictably, such institutions were usually unwelcome to practitioners in those areas, who saw Lilley Smith's dispensaries as rivals to their own incomes.

Even before opening the self-supporting dispensary at Southam, Lilley Smith had founded an Eye and Ear Infirmary in this small market town, based on J. C. Saunders's establishment of 1805. It was essentially a miniature version of the great eighteenth-century voluntary hospitals, in that subscribers could nominate patients, vice presidents paid five guineas a year and only those too poor to pay, for whom the parish contributed, were admitted free. Patients, however, were expected to pay for the cost of their accommodation at 8d. a day for a man, 6d. for a woman and 4d. for a child; there were fourteen beds. The Eye and Ear Infirmary opened in 1818 and occupied a handsome building 'in the Gothic style ... on an elevated and healthy situation, and ... fitted out in the most commodious manner'. Lilley Smith was convinced that many poor people, suffering from diseases of the eyes and ears, received inadequate treatment and their general health then deteriorated, often obliging them to become dependant on the parish. Unlike the voluntary hospitals, sufferers were admitted daily and Lilley Smith also visited neighbouring communities to see patients after they had been discharged.

During the years 1818–57 an average of 315 patients a year were treated at the infirmary, ranging from a maximum of 395 in 1821–2 and a minimum of 263 in 1824–5. The published list of eye conditions treated in 1831–2 suggests that common ophthalmic diseases predominated (the majority noted as 'inflammation') and that most needed long-term attention. Not surprisingly, the Poor Law Commissioner, C. P. Villiers, commented strongly in favour of Lilley Smith's work, because his dispensaries enabled the free, independent class to provide for themselves, 'whenever properly encouraged', and thus avoid pauperism. Villiers noted that out of Southam's population of 1,161, 681 were labourers and of these 145 were regular paupers and a further 400 had received medical relief. However, after the dispensary was established, 170 had become free members and were no longer attended by the parish surgeon. Villiers also expressed 'unmixed satisfaction' at the equally striking figures for Birmingham, Aston and Derby.

Unfortunately, after Lilley Smith's death in 1859 at the age of seventy-one the Eye and Ear Infirmary did not thrive, and it was incorporated into the Warneford

Hospital at Leamington Spa in 1872. Towards the end of his life Lilley Smith supported some bizarre and extreme socio-religious causes that detracted from his status as a medical pioneer. His real achievements, however, were his novel suggestions for bringing medical attention to the poor yet avoiding the stigma of pauperism and entry into the workhouse. His obituary notice commented that the poor wept at his death. He is commemorated in Southam with a monumental urn on the site of the dispensary cottage; the Eye and Ear Infirmary is now an hotel.

Specialist eye institutions continued to be established throughout the nineteenth century, some only short-lived, so that there were fifteen founded in the years 1834–61, eight in 1866–80 and ten in 1881–9, as well as nine in London (1804–57), a real indication of the demand for ophthalmic care in the country as a whole. Specialist institutions continued to multiply in the nineteenth century, many filling a genuine need, such as those for treating consumption, children's diseases and fever. However, some were certainly established as a means of practice-building and in response to scarce posts in established hospitals, condemned by *The Lancet* as 'this rampant evil of over-weening specialism' in 1863, and some infirmaries did not allow their physicians and surgeons to work in a special hospital. Viewed from a distance, however, specialist hospitals provided an opportunity for improvements and innovations in medical treatments that were not possible in the great contemporary general hospitals.

Patients admitted to Birmingham Hospital, 6–13 November 1779

Patient	Recommended by	Age	Parish	Distemper	Discharged	How dischd
Sarah Page	Samuel Tutin	20	B'ham	3m sore leg	1 Jan	cured
Wm Elstone	Thomas Gil	25	B'ham	4m paralytic	8 Jan	relieved
Sarah Hodgkins	Revd Riland	21	Sutton	9m hectica	4 Dec	cured
Mary Newby	Sam Hammond	23	B'ham	6w sore legs	4 Dec	cured
Sarah Lewis	Josiah Pratt	24	W.Brom	1yr ulcers	29 Jan	cured
Eliz Simnett	Joseph Townsend	44	B'ham	2yr sore leg	4 Dec	cured
Ann Pickering*	W.J.Banner	22	B'ham	3m consumption	11 Dec	cured
Jn Chaulton*	Edward Jones	2	B'ham	scrophula	11 Dec	cured
Mary Thornton*	William Bratt	16	B'ham	hectica	11 Dec	cured
John Martin*	Thomas Lawrence	21	W. Brom	9m consumption	11 Dec	cured
Ralph Hammersley*	J. Bentley	21	B'ham	1m rheumatic	11 Dec	cured
Eliz Moseley*	Jonathon Collison	12	B'ham	1yr worms	11 Dec	cured
Sarah Carless*	Joseph Kendall	30	W Brom	1m cough	27 Nov	cured
Wm Partridge*	Accident	12	n.s.	fractured elbow	8 Dec	cured
Ann Hughes*	Edmund Hector	40	B'ham	sore leg	1 Jan	cured
Sarah Davis*	John Ryland	60	n.s	fever	18 Dec	cured
John Bennett*	Daniel Hodgkins	33	B'ham	gravel	1 Jan	cured
Obadiah Cashmore	John Townsend	18	Cradley	1 yr lame hip	4 Dec	relieved
Esau Turner	William Holden	64	B'ham 10m	sore legs	12 Feb	cured
Th Harrison	John Fothergill	28	Wootton	2m fever	1 Jan	relieved

Patient	Recommended by	Age	Parish	Distemper	Discharged	How dischd
Eliz Lambert	Atherstone Overseers	27	Mancetter	3yr white swelling+	12 Feb	cured
Richard Evans	Accident?	15	Aston	ulcered leg	18 Dec	cured

* out patients
+ amputated above the knee, 25 November

Physicians:	6–12 November John Ash;
	13–20 November William Withering
Surgeons:	6–12 November George Kennedy
	13–20 November Jeremiah Vaux and Robert Ward

Birmingham Archives, hospital admissions register, 1779–88

Note
n.s. = not stated

State of the General Infirmary at Hereford, 1798–99

A GENERAL ABSTRACT of the STATE of the PATIENTS,
from the First Establishment, 26th of March, 1776, to 25th March, 1799.

IN-PATIENTS		OUT-PATIENTS	
Admitted, as by former Reports	3553		5792
Ditto, from March 25, 1798, to			
March 25, 1799	145–3698		165–5957
Cured	2043		3778
Relieved	210		256
For Misbehaviour	92		16
Discharged At their own Request	63		9
Run away	1		
Improper	15		1
Incurable	21		7
Not coming on a Vacancy	17	Non-Attendance	1491
Dead	175	Known to be Dead	178
Made Out-Patients	1041	Made In-Patients	261
	3678		5927

Remaining in the House, March 25, 1799 20 – 3698 On the Books 30 – 5957
Total of In and Out-Patients to the 25th of March, 1799 – 9655.

N.B. *On account of the Number of Surgical Cases constantly in the Hospital, requiring a large Quantity of Lint, and Cloth for Rollers, &c. old Linen will be esteemed a valuable Present to the Charity.*

Privately owned

This is a typical annual report distributed to hospital subscribers, including their names, contributions and an abstract of the financial accounts for the year. During the year covered by the accounts, £506 13s. 9d. was received and £549 15s. spent. There were 195 annual subscriptions for the year, including 48 from clergy, ranging from £10 10s. to a guinea.

ASYLUMS AND PRISONS

BLUNT'S ASYLUM WIGSTON MAGNA
The Insane will meet with a comfortable Home, and have every possible Effort
used for their Relief and Recovery. Patients of all Ranks are treated with
Humanity and Kindness; the extent and situation of this Asylum admits of
suitable Accommodation being assigned to everyone, which entirely prevents
any unpleasant interference with each other

Warwick Advertiser, 17 March 1810

Of all the varieties of medical care, the services provided for the mentally ill are
the most diverse, difficult to trace and analyse, especially in the constantly-shift-
ing views of insanity that prevailed across two centuries. Different generations
held divergent opinions over what constituted insanity, how far the eccentric
and the simple-minded should be included and whether provision should be
institutional or private, coercive or liberal. As in all other aspects of medical
care, money was a crucial factor. The simple, poor 'village idiot' figure could be
maintained, long-term, by the parish, while carrying out unskilled tasks such as
scaring birds or picking stones in the countryside, sweeping streets or holding
horses' heads in the town. As the population both grew and became more indus-
trialised by the later eighteenth century, mental illness afflicted noticeably more
people overall, and some conditions were the result of a wider definition of
insanity while others were directly attributable to new, dangerous occupations
and substances, especially lead and mercury that caused brain damage. However,
this was a problem of which the medical profession was only slowly becoming
aware, in spite of the works of Ramazzini and Thackrah.

Even in the seventeenth century, when the humoral theory of disease reigned,
there were mental patients in some basic categories that were to change little,
those who were clinically depressed ('the melancholics') and those who were
physically violent, both to themselves and to others ('the maniacs'). There were
sufferers from what are now recognisable and treatable conditions, including
schizophrenia, epilepsy and hormonal imbalance, who were almost automatically
consigned to an institution, public or private. There were also, at all periods,
patients who were insane as a result of their lifestyles, suffering from tertiary
syphilis, alcoholism or drug abuse, and these too would be incarcerated. The

most affluent, whatever the diagnosis, could be kept in their family home, under personal restraint, the Mrs Rochester solution fictionalised in *Jane Eyre*, but practised for only a handful of very wealthy but unmanageable individuals in the eighteenth and nineteenth centuries. Such 'single lunatics' were never the concern of authority and we know of them only from random personal accounts. Thus the Revd James Clegg recorded in his diary how he lodged Mrs Elizabeth Touchet, described as 'raving', in November 1739 until she became too unmanageable and was sent home.

The tension between custody and cure became unavoidable by the early nineteenth century, as did the sheer overall number of paupers in England by the 1830s, of whom mental patients, even if an unchanging proportion, grew remorselessly. Enhanced life expectancy, for the inmates as for the rest of society, also added to the problem. In addition, there were new concepts of what constituted madness, with melancholy fashionable by the late eighteenth century as a mark of refinement and sensitivity in artistic circles and, for example, three well-known poets of the eighteenth century, William Collins, William Cowper and Christopher Smart, were all confined as lunatics. There was also a growing belief that institutions should cure inmates and return them as useful citizens to the community, not simply keep them shut away for life. Lunacy was accepted as a cause for annulling a marriage and, after 1912, if incurable, for divorce. As early as 1628 being in the state of *non compos mentis* had been defined and, since insane persons lacked intent to commit a crime, they could not be liable for an offence, even murder. For female criminals there were special physiological reasons for madness, including lactation insanity or puerperal mania, suppressed menstruation and menopausal symptoms, as well as a heredity factor. Lunacy in the eighteenth century was clearly controlled by the magistrates rather than the medical profession.

From 1760 insanity was acknowledged as a defence plea in court and in 1800 (40 Geo. III, *c*. 94) the Criminal Lunatics' Act was passed which permitted a verdict of 'not guilty' by reason of insanity. By the 1840s, medical witnesses with new expertise were increasingly important in the courts, including John Conolly, and 1843 saw the introduction of the McNaughtan Rules setting out precise legal criteria by which to judge how far the insane were criminally responsible. The later nineteenth-century label of 'criminally insane' created a further category of high-security institutions, such as Rampton and Broadmoor. The Mental Deficiency Act of 1913, following the Report of the Royal Commission of Inquiry into the Care and Control of the Feeble-Minded (1904–8), pronounced that those who suffered from 'moral imbecility' should go to special institutions and not to prisons. Medical teaching on psychiatry, however, lagged far behind practical experience, but in 1823 Sir Alexander Morison MD began a course of lectures in London and Edinburgh and two years later published his *Outlines of Lectures on Mental Diseases*, which ran to five editions. In this, he included illustrations of the insane and in 1838 produced *Physiognomy of Mental Diseases*, the first English text on this topic. He was later consulting physician to Bethlem and the asylums at Hanwell and Springfield.

Evidence for how the insane were treated before the mid-eighteenth century is, perhaps predictably, extremely sparse, and survives really only for patients sent to institutions such as Bethlem and a minority in private care. However, something had to be done for those who were physically dangerous, to themselves or to others, pauper or prosperous, and scattered references suggest that there were madhouses for such patients, as well as the boarding-out of individuals in private clerical or medical households. In Wiltshire there was an asylum as early as 1615 at Box, one at Glastonbury in 1656, at Newcastle upon Tyne in 1686 and at Bilston in c. 1700. Parish officials were also obliged to make arrangements for their lunatic paupers, although such references, like the accounts themselves, in seventeenth-century Overseers' ledgers are very rare. However, in May 1698 the parish of Kenilworth made provisions for a poor lunatic, Richard Knight, including a meeting of 'the neighbours ...to consult what course to take about him'. He was fed, clothed, lodged and attended, as well as being pursued when he outran his keeper. The cost to the parish was £3 17s. 11d., as well as £10 for boarding Knight in a madhouse run by Mr Bellcher for twelve months. Knight died after a year there. In 1714 an Act was passed (12 Anne, c. 23) to distinguish pauper lunatics from disorderly persons, rogues and vagabonds, allowing two magistrates to confine the 'furiously mad', who were no longer to be whipped as a punishment. The Vagrancy Act thirty years later (17 Geo. II, c. 5) charged parishes with 'curing such Persons during such Restraint', the first reference in law to treating the insane, and have them confined in 'some secure place', if necessary in chains.

The most famous, or notorious, of all British asylums, however, was Bethlem, founded in the thirteenth century by a Crusader returning home and originally the priory of St Mary of Bethlehem. At the Dissolution, Henry VIII presented Bethlem to the mayor and corporation of London as a refuge for sufferers who had no friends or family to pay for them. In 1675–6 a large new hospital was built for 120 inmates, designed by Robert Hooke, the City Surveyor, in 'single pile' style at a cost of £17,000 at Moorfields, its combination of long corridors and rows of cells a model for later institutions when secure confinement was critical. Its new, sophisticated architecture made it one of the contemporary tourist attractions in the capital, frequently depicted in engravings, with its own gardens and bathing place for the inmates. A new wing for incurables was added in 1723. As well as royal and aristocratic visitors, such as the Duke of Monmouth, Bethlem was of considerable interest to practitioners, so that the diaries of James Yonge of Plymouth (in 1678) and Richard Kaye of Bury (1743–4), both surgeons, were among those who noted their visits there.

By the mid-eighteenth century, in an age of enhanced sensibility, visiting Bethlem as an entertainment became increasingly unacceptable. Formerly it had been considered an instructive and moral experience to view the insane, who exemplified the wages of sin and indulgence. The Bethlem Governors were undecided about the merits of allowing visitors, who undoubtedly contributed to the charity's funds, with about £400 a year placed in the poor's box and the prospect that future bequests might be made. Disorderly visitors (including Methodist preachers) were proving particularly troublesome and individual admission tickets were required, signed by a Governor, after 1777, when Bethlem was financially secure and less dependent on visitors' donations. Undoubtedly, increasing public squeamishness was a factor and caused the insane to be isolated from society.

A prominent medical family, the Monros, ran Bethlem from 1728 until 1833, although daily care was always in the hands of the keepers. When John Howard visited in 1788 there were a hundred incurables, half of them women; their relatives paid only 2s. 6d. a week for their maintenance. He reported that 'the patients communicate with one another from the top to the bottom of the house, so that there is no separation of the calm and quiet from the noisy and turbulent, except those who are chained in their cells'. For 270 rooms on four floors there was only one privy, 'very offensive', and yet the rooms were quite clean. The regime was harsh and coercive; while manacles can be clearly seen in Hogarth's illustration of 1735 (Figure 6.1), purgatives and emetics were standard treatments. Undoubtedly, George III's five attacks of insanity brought increased awareness of the condition and the plight of all sufferers, especially with the publication of detailed parliamentary reports on his health and therapy. However, even before the king's illness, another lunatic asylum, St Luke's, had been built in London, in Windmill Street, Upper Moorfields in 1751; its architect was George Dance, senior. It was replaced in 1789 by a building in Old Street for

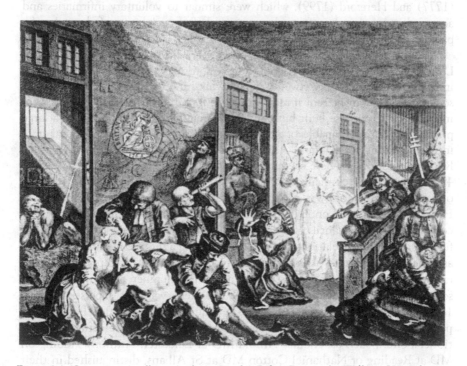

Figure 6.1 'Scene in a madhouse', plate viii of *A Rake's Progress* by William Hogarth.

which Dance's son was the architect. Its founder was William Battie, the author of *A Treatise on Madness* (1757) and a critic of the Bethlem methods, who taught psychiatry to his medical students at St Luke's. Incurable inmates paid 5s. a week. Here occupational therapy was used and inmates had a more humanised existence, with less coercion and bleeding, although wards were unheated. Paying spectators were not allowed and family visits were limited to half an hour in length. Intended for the 'middling' class of lunatic, by 1780 the original building had some 110 inmates, of whom thirty were incurable.

The eighteenth century saw a dramatic change in reactions to the insane, so that, although it was acceptable early in the century for Pope and Swift to satirise the lunatic and for the inmates at Bethlem to be viewed as a genteel public entertainment, such attitudes were altered completely by the last decade, when The Retreat at York marked an outlook of kindness and cure, rather than punitive treatment, incarceration and mockery. There were, in the eighteenth and nineteenth centuries, three distinct categories of institutions that would admit mental patients: the private madhouse, the charitable institution and the public asylum, although none was entirely exclusive. Thus, the private madhouse would admit paupers, paid for by their parish, as well as affluent patients, while the charitable institution, such as Norwich Bethel, took in all lunatics irrespective of their financial circumstances, as at Newcastle upon Tyne (1765), Manchester (1766), York (1777) and Hereford (1799), which were similar to voluntary infirmaries and accepted inmates on benefactors' recommendations as 'objects of charity' or by paying fees.

As early as 1714 Defoe noted that there were fifteen private madhouses in London and Parry-Jones has shown the extraordinary growth in their numbers in the eighteenth century (twenty in Warwickshire, for example), to which all social classes might be sent if funds could be found. Early private asylums were invariably not purpose-built but converted premises, such as an inn or a large private house, and capable of accommodating only a fairly small number of inmates, so that, for example, Anthony Addington had only eight or ten at his Reading madhouse. These establishments after an Act of 1774 (14 Geo. III, *c.* 49) were inspected annually and licensed in each county by Quarter Sessions; one of the inspectors was a local medical practitioner (Baron Dimsdale in Hertfordshire, John Conolly in Middlesex, for example). However, the Act covered the circumstances of only private inmates, not of paupers, and wrongful incarceration by relations was at least as strong a motive in passing this Act as concern for patients' physical welfare. From the inspectors' reports, although rare archive survivals, it is possible to assess the number of occupants, their social class and medical condition. This system was not superseded until 1828, when an Act (9 Geo. IV, *c.* 41) required Home Office licensing of private asylums. Until then, many madhouse proprietors were actually practitioners, often, such as Thomas Arnold MD at Leicester, Anthony Addington MD at Reading or Nathaniel Cotton MD at St Albans, distinguished in their profession.

However, madhouse-keeping could be a family business, as with the Harrises at Hook Norton, and women often ran asylums, although invariably they were the wives or daughters of the original proprietors. The essentially business nature of running madhouses may be seen in press advertisements for their services. When John Thurstan, surgeon-apothecary of Bilston, died in 1756, 'the whole care and management' of his lunatics came under the care of John Vernon, his former apprentice and journeyman, who was also a local surgeon's brother and a physician's nephew. Inmates were often from a wide catchment area, so that, for example, Vernon advertised his Staffordshire asylum in Worcestershire. His rival in the same locality, Joseph Proud, in the same week announced in *Aris's Birmingham Gazette* that he had taken over his late father's asylum, which was:

> A large and convenient house ... in a retired and airy situation, with a garden walled round, for the safety and privacy of his patients, with a cold bath upon the premises, which in many cases is very necessary in that dreadful malady; the experience he has had by assisting his father, Samuel Proud, who, for upwards of fifty years, had kept a house for lunatics, and is well known in most parts of this kingdom, for the many and great cures he has perform'd in that disorder, has qualified him to treat that malady, in all its various appearances, with propriety and judgment: All persons who are committed to his care may depend upon being treated with the greatest humanity and care.

Wherever lunatics were confined, security was a vital factor and contemporary newspapers advertised when inmates, usually harmless, went missing from work-houses or asylums.

The charges for residence in an asylum were considerable, especially as the patient might remain as an inmate for many months or even years. Fees varied only slightly between institutions but significantly between paupers and non-poor. In London rates were higher than in the provinces, with £13 or £15 for six months (10s. or 12s. a week) in the early nineteenth century at Hoxton and Bethnal Green asylums. In the country, 7s. or 8s. a week was usually charged for a pauper, but even so the drain on the Overseers' funds was substantial when a parishioner was incarcerated for many years. Thus, an Allesley man was at Proud's asylum from 1777 until 1805 at a total cost to his parish of £331 8s. He was then finally moved to the House of Industry at nearby Meriden.

Some madhouses were, however, prepared to undercut the local rates, so that in 1787, when Proud was charging two guineas on entrance and £30 a year, his rival, George Chadwick at Lichfield, required only one guinea and £17 a year for an inmate.

Prosperous patients, however, paid considerably more than paupers, and Mary Lamb, the poet's sister, placed in an Islington asylum after she murdered her mother in 1796, had accommodation of a better grade than at the standard £50 a year, with a personal servant to attend her. Apart from the basic charge of between one and four guineas a week, there were extra expenses for laundry, often for medicines, linen, clothes and services such as hairdressing or sewing. Private patients, however, occupied single rooms, had superior food and a better ratio of staff to inmates; they usually had no contact with any paupers in the madhouse. By the early nineteenth century Warburton's house at Hackney apparently charged the Duke of Atholl's son £1,500 a year as a patient in this extremely large institution with nearly five hundred inmates, most of whom were paupers. All asylums recorded a very low rate of cured patients, although John Blount, a Warwick surgeon-apothecary, claimed in his advertisement in 1810 that, out of sixteen in his care, ten patients were 'restored to Society', two or three were 'irrecoverable' and the rest convalescent.

No matter how expensive private accommodation at such asylums may have been, at the very highest level, for the care provided by the most famous royal mad doctors, Willis and Monro, charges were significantly higher. The fees for one such patient, Edward 5th Lord Leigh (1742–86), are recorded in detail. As a child he inherited a grand Warwickshire house, Stoneleigh Abbey, on the death of his father in 1749 and spent lavishly on its further improvements. In 1765 he became ill when in France and the estate ledgers show extensive medical expenses for the rest of his life, to John Monro and particularly to Francis Willis. In 1768 Monro was paid £49 7s. for visiting Lord Leigh seventeen times in London and six times in Warwickshire, but after 1771 treatment was provided by Willis. Francis Willis since 1760 had a private asylum at Dunston (later moving to Greatford) in Lincolnshire, where he charged Leigh £1,260 a year (£105 a month). Lord Leigh was at Willis's house for nearly three years, but in 1773 a Commission in Lunacy was obtained to administer the considerable Leigh estate. The local press noted that 'his Lordship was of unsound mind, and had not for several years been capable of managing his very noble estate and fortune'. Arrangements were then made for Lord Leigh to live at Stoneleigh under restraint, where he had a resident surgeon-apothecary to attend him for the remaining thirteen years of his life. The man appointed was James Butler, whose brother was agent to the estate, and who had been apprenticed locally in 1744.

Later famous for treating George III, Willis was nicknamed 'the Duplicate Doctor' because he was qualified both as a cleric and as a medical practitioner. He was very secretive about his methods of treating the insane and, as he declared that he kept no case notes, information about his patients is very erratic, to be gleaned only from other sources. Thus we know that he attended and boarded Sanderson Miller, the gentleman-architect, in the 1770s only from the patient's family papers. Willis's 'piercing gaze' added to his reputation as possessing magical healing powers. However, he claimed that nine out of ten of his patients were cured and he was later awarded a very large pension for attending George III.

However, a concern for the mentally afflicted, as for those who suffered physically, stirred eighteenth-century society and a handful of charitable asylums were established in the provinces as a result. The earliest of these was at

Norwich, founded by a clergy widow, Mary Chapman, in 1713 for 'distrest lunaticks', although not for 'such as are fools or idiots from their birth'. At her death in 1724 her estate of £3,513 was invested for income to run the asylum; there were usually between twenty and thirty inmates, the majority female. By the late eighteenth century the Norwich Bethel had fifty beds attended by two salaried physicians and seventy beds by 1845.

Other charitable asylums were not founded until over fifty years later, with institutions at Manchester, Newcastle upon Tyne, York and Hereford all established in the eighteenth century, as well as The Retreat at York, which was exclusively for insane Quakers. The asylum at Manchester, staffed by the three physicians and three surgeons who served the main infirmary, next to which it was sited, was opened in 1766 initially for twenty-two patients, but held a hundred by the end of the century. A physician visited once a week. Sightseers were not allowed and the sexes were segregated. Treatment was free, but patients paid for everything else at a rate of 7s. a week for paupers, but 10s. for the non-poor. John Ferriar MD published his *Medical Histories and Reflections* (1792 and 1795) on his work there, advocating mildness and conciliation towards the insane.

At Newcastle upon Tyne plans were made in 1765 for a charitable public asylum in Bath Lane for lunatics from the counties of Northumberland and Durham and it opened two years later, designed by the local architect, William Newton, at the beginning of his career. From its early days the Newcastle Common Council gave financial support (ten guineas a year) but within a few years the asylum was licensed to the town's leading physician, John Hall, who already had his own private madhouse in Newcastle. In the first half century of its existence, the asylum claimed to have treated 402 patients, of whom 158 were cured, forty-nine were better, sixty-nine left 'by their own desire', sixty-seven died and, in 1817, fifty-nine were still inmates. The asylum was virtually reconstructed in 1824 by another local architect, John Dobson, but was demolished in c. 1866.

The York Asylum, designed for fifty-four inmates, 'either parish poor or belonging to distressed and indigent families', opened in 1774 after public appeals, begun in 1772, raised £5,000. The architect was John Carr, whose other commissions in the city had included the Assize Courts, the Female Prison and Fairfax House. There were initially ten patients each paying 8s. a week in 1774, with a guinea deposit to offset the charge of a funeral. Categories of patients denied admission were the incurables from other asylums, epileptics, idiots, the pregnant and those suffering from venereal disease, all also generally excluded from other institutions. A decade later the governors decided to accept a few wealthy patients to help provide funds for the poorer inmates and Dr Alexander Hunter increasingly ran the asylum as 'a house of retirement for persons of condition only', who paid £1 a week plus medical fees. In 1794 the asylum could publish a notice in the local press that between 1777 and 1793 a total of 822 patients had been admitted, of whom 404 were cured, 193 released, seventy-nine incurable and sixty-four dead. There were then seventy-four inmates, twenty-four of whom were poor. The scandal of a female Quaker's death there in 1791, accusations of false accounting, serious overcrowding (160 patients in premises built for only fifty-four) and a fire resulted in widespread reforms, including the physician receiving a salary instead of patients' fees. The House of Commons Select Committee Report in 1815 noted only seven keepers for 199 inmates there, whereas at the York Retreat the ratio was one for every ten inmates. In 1828 new accommodation was added for fourteen violent patients. Wealthy inmates were presumably affected by the asylum's tarnished reputation, for by 1815 twelve private madhouses had opened in the York area. The situation eased when the West Riding Asylum opened at Wakefield in 1818 and by 1847 paupers were excluded when the North and East Riding Asylum was built at Clifton, near York, for 144 patients. In 1906 the city's own lunatic asylum was opened and accommodated up to four hundred patients until 1940.

The fourth of these eighteenth-century charitable lunatic asylums in the provinces was established at Hereford in 1799, sited next to the General Hospital on the banks of the River Wye. The infirmary had opened there in 1776 with fifty-five beds and a year later a charitable lunatic asylum was proposed:

> Whereas, from the miserable state of the distemper itself, as well as from its rendering the objects of it, not only burdens but terrors to Society ...
> It is to be observed that the security and cure of Lunatics in private families is almost impracticable. And such have been the abuses of private mad houses, through the ignorance and venality of the keepers, that the Legislature, in the 14th year of the present reign, passed an act to obviate them; but this act, as yet, has been little attended to.

The asylum was intended for all social classes who were 'unfortunate victims of this terrible distemper'. Unhappily, the project was delayed for over twenty years, and it was not until 1799 that the infirmary Governors had collected £1,481 and 'adopted the Proposal of extending the Usefulness of this Charity by adding an Asylum for the Reception of Lunaticks', although financially separate from the infirmary. Twenty patients were to be admitted initially with an experienced keeper, who had formerly worked at Bethlem. However, he was unsatisfactory and two years later the asylum was effectively privatised and leased to a local surgeon. Abuses reported there under a new proprietor, William Gilliland MD, caused a Parliamentary Select Committee to investigate in 1839. It was alleged that paupers were admitted with improperly signed certificates and, although poor record-keeping seems to have been a common misdemeanour in asylums, cruelty towards inmates was the real complaint of mismanagement at Hereford. In addition, there was overcrowding, patients were unclassified and religious services were not held. Restraint was widely practised and Gilliland admitted that he used the cold bath both as a treatment and to punish inmates, but also quoted letters from grateful patients cured by this form of therapy. The asylum's Visitors reported to Quarter Sessions that it 'was not in that state, either as relates to ventilation, to classification, to employment, to moral treatment, to recreation and religious consolation for convalescents, which they would wish to prevail'. However, although refused a licence by the county magistrates, the city's JPs granted one. The asylum closed in 1853 and a public institution was opened at Burghill in 1872, which had eleven wards for 550 inmates. The county asylum ran its own hundred-acre farm, which helped keep patients' costs modest and in 1902 its death-rate was the lowest recorded in English asylums.

The Retreat, built at Heslington, near York, set in twelve acres, opened in June 1796, was unique as an asylum exclusively for Quakers. Its existence, the result of the ill-treatment and mysterious death of a Quaker girl in York Asylum in 1791 after only a short time there, was initiated by a local Quaker, William Tuke (1732–1822), a tea and coffee merchant, a year later. Purpose-built at a cost of £3,869, The Retreat lacked the usual barred windows and perimeter walls. The architect was John Bevans of Plaistow, a Quaker, who also designed several meeting houses for the Society of Friends. The Retreat had accommodation for thirty inmates and in the first year fifteen were admitted, for whom charges were only 4s. or 8s. a week, reduced for a stay of six months or longer. Thomas Fowler MD, recently physician at Stafford Infirmary, but originally from York, was in charge of this 'mild system of treatment' and the matron was Mrs Katherine Jepson, who had formerly worked for Edward Long Fox at Cleeve. There were sixty-six inmates in The Retreat by 1812 and ninety-four by 1828; wealthy patients paid from one to five guineas a week. The whole regime was based on regarding inmates as part of a family, living and eating together, with occupational therapy such as gardening, chess and handicrafts. The Retreat also pioneered the first use of animals in a therapeutic setting, for patients were encouraged to care for small animals and poultry to learn self-control by 'having dependent on them creatures weaker than themselves'. Patients were to be treated respectfully and restraint was not to be used. Rather than starving the insane to keep them physically weak and more manageable, Tuke fed the inmates well, noting that a large evening meal and good porter to drink would make them sleep soundly and avoid the use of opium. In May 1813 Samuel Tuke, the founder's grandson, published his *Description of the Retreat*, detailing treatments, cases and design; it was widely seen as a criticism of the York Asylum. General disquiet about the York Asylum's conditions resulted in the setting up of a Parliamentary Select Committee in 1815, to which, at the age of eighty-three, William Tuke gave evidence.

A claim to being the first institution, earlier than The Retreat, for humane treatment of the insane was made by Edward Long Fox (Figure 6.2), also a Quaker, at Cleeve Hill, near Bristol, a small private house owned by the Society of Friends, which he took over in 1794 as an asylum. A year later he was advertising that the premises were enlarged, not exclusively for Quakers, and that his regime was non-coercive. In 1804 his rival to The Retreat was the newly-built Brislington House, near Bristol, for seventy patients, 'which is believed to have been nearly, if not quite, the first private asylum that had ever been built

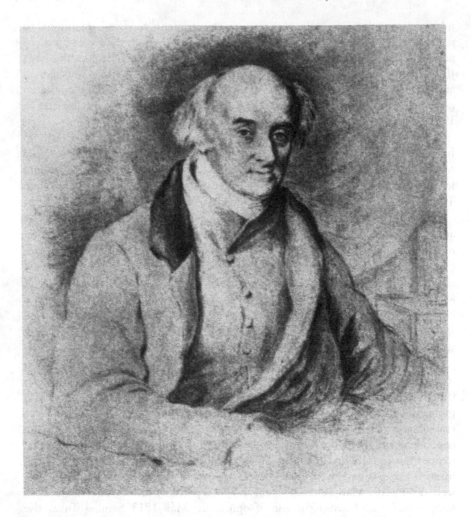

Figure 6.2 Dr Edward Long Fox of Brislington, portrait by an unknown artist. By kind permission of the Frenchay Tuckett Society.

purposely for the reception of the insane'. His sons, also practitioners who later ran the establishment, wrote of its facilities in considerable detail in 1836, emphasising the various categories of accommodation for different social classes, with violent inmates segregated and regular Anglican divine service for patients in their own chapel. At Brislington, 'all personal coercion [was] suspended', while 'bodily exercise' included bowls, cricket and football, as well as music and a library for 'mental recreation'. Fox believed in the merits of both hypnotism and sea bathing. The patient statistics for Brislington in the 1830s and 40s show a minority of paupers, a very low rate of suicides and deaths, as well as a predominance of men over women inmates; a fifth of all patients suffered from melancholia. The palatial Brislington House is now a nursing home.

By the early nineteenth century a reliable sign of government concern about any social phenomenon was the setting up of a Parliamentary Select Committee and in 1807 one was formed to investigate the state of pauper and criminal lunatics in England and Wales, their numbers and where they were housed. Although all the detailed evidence is extremely interesting, the most striking proposal to come from this Select Committee was the plan for dividing the kingdom into sixteen districts 'for the Erection of Lunatic Asylums', each for up to three hundred inmates. Lancashire and Yorkshire were to have one each, while the other counties were in groups of two to four for their proposed asylums, which would be situated at appropriate regional centres, such as Nottingham, Exeter and Canterbury; each district had a population of about half a million. An Act for the Better Care and Maintenance of Lunatics (48 Geo.III, c. 96) was passed in the following year, giving counties the power to build asylums, which they were remarkably reluctant to do. In 1815 a further Act (55 Geo. III, c. 46) allowed counties to borrow money for this purpose. In fact, only eight were built by 1825 and, even twenty years after the passing of the 1808 Act, only ten out of fifty-two counties had actually done so. Indeed, under the permissive Act most county lunatic asylums were in the traditionally rural counties (Norfolk, Lincoln, Cornwall, Gloucester, Suffolk, Dorset and Kent), although Lancashire and the West Riding of Yorkshire, heavily populated areas, were among the first to open county asylums, followed by Bedfordshire. Staffordshire was a leader in building a county pauper lunatic asylum in 1818 for up to 120 inmates. Its architect, Joseph Potter, was a local man and the venture attracted considerable criticism, especially at the expense to the county. The weekly charge for patients was reduced when neighbouring counties contracted to supply numbers of paupers; Birmingham sent thirty, while Worcestershire inmates were admitted at 11s. a week. To save money, many Staffordshire paupers were moved there from the local private madhouses kept by Proud and Bakewell. Interestingly, a local landowner, Lord Hatherton of Teddesley, visited the new asylum in November 1818, when, he noted, there were thirty-three lunatics. Among these, 'One man fancied himself the Keeper of the Asylum, and told us it was no use talking to any of the men, for they had not an ounce of sense'. Overcrowding became acute in the 1820s, so that the asylum had a hundred inmates by 1821 but 150 by 1825; a peak of 186 was reached in September 1828. The majority of lunatics, however, still remained in private institutions until the Act became mandatory in 1845 and most county lunatic asylums were built after this date (Table 6.1). However, nineteenth-century public subscriptions had also established asylums at Oxford (the Warneford, 1821), Liverpool (1828), Northampton (1836) and Coton Hill, Staffordshire (1854) in addition to the pauper county asylums.

In 1807 the pressure for pauper places was such that St Luke's, capable of accommodating about a hundred inmates, had seven hundred applications when a single vacancy occurred. The cost to a county of a purpose-built asylum was

Table 6.1 County Lunatic Asylums in England

	Place	Date		Architect
Bedfordshire	Bedford	1809–12	1825 enlarged	John Wing, jun
	Arlesley	1857	cost £114,831	George F. Jones
Berkshire	Cholsey	1867–70		C.H.Howell
Buckinghamshire	Stone	1849–53		T. H. Wyatt &
				D. Brandon
Cambridgeshire	Fulbourn	1853–8	cost £40,000	George F. Jones
Cheshire	Chester	1827–29		William Cole
Cornwall	Bodmin	1817–20		John Foulston
Cumberland &	Carlisle	1862		J. A. Cory
Westmorland				
Derbyshire	Mickleover	1849–51		Henry Duesbury
Devonshire	Exminster	1842–45		Charles Fowler
Dorset	Forston	1832		
	Charminster	1859–63		H.E.Kendall, jun
Durham	Sedgefield	1859		John Howison
Essex	Brentwood	1849		H.E.Kendall, jun
Gloucestershire	Gloucester	1813–23		William Stark
	Coney Hill	1884		John Giles & ... Gough
Hampshire	Funtley	1852	cost £33,786	J. Harris
Herefordshire	Burghill	1868–71		Robert Griffiths
Hertfordshire	St Albans	1899		G. T. Hine
Kent	Maidstone	1830–33		John Whichcord, sen
Lancashire	Lancaster	1812–16		Thomas Standen
	Prestwich	1851		Willliam Moseley
	Rainhill	1847–51		H. L. Elmes & W.
				Moseley
Leicestershire	Leicester	1837		William Parsons
Lincolnshire	Bracebridge	1848–9	tender of	... Hamilton & Thos
	Heath		£32,870	Perry
Middlesex	Hanwell	1829–31		William Alderson
	Colney Hatch	1847,1849–51		Samuel W. Daukes
Norfolk	Thorpe	1811–14	cost £40,000	Francis Stone
Nottinghamshire	Sneinton	1810–12		Richard Ingleman
Oxfordshire	Littlemore	1844–6		R. N.Clark
Shropshire	Shelton	1843–5		G. G. Scott & W. L.
				Moffatt
Somerset	Wells	1845–8		Scott & Moffatt
Staffordshire	St George's	1818		Joseph Potter
	Burntwood	1864		William L. Moffatt
Suffolk	Melton	1828		
Surrey	Wandsworth	1838–41		William Moseley
	Brookwood	1862–7		C. H. Howell
	Banstead	1873		S. H. Parnell
	Netherne	1901–9		G. T. Hine
Sussex	Haywards Heath	1856–9		H. E. Kendall, jun

Place		Date		Architect
Warwickshire	Hatton	1849–52	cost £68,000	J. Harris & F. J. Francis
Wiltshire	Roundway, Devizes	1848–51		T. H.Wyatt
Worcestershire	Powick	1847–52		Hamilton & Medland
Yorkshire	Wakefield	1816–18		C. Watson & James P. Pritchett
	Hull	1879–83		Smith & Broderick
	Clifton	1845–7		G. G. Scott & W. L. Moffatt
	Sheffield Middlewood	1872	cost £80,000	Bernard Hartley
	Menston	1888		J. Vickers Edwards

considerable and the distinguished architect John Nash, who had prepared (but never executed) plans for asylums at Hereford, Exeter and Gloucester, told the 1807 Committee that a pauper institution in London for only fifty inmates would cost £7,760. Among the earliest county asylums was Nottingham's, situated at Sneinton, and opened in 1812; it was built on the Bethlem pattern at a cost of £20,000 to hold fifty-six patients. For all categories of lunatics, weekly charges ranged from 9s. to three guineas or more. A contemporary visitor there noted:

> Every patient has a distinct lodging room; & the provisions for air & ventilation are excellent; there are six spacious airing courts for the patients to walk in; and a large garden …This is certainly a place where any person might send their friends with satisfaction.

Although Tuke's regime had admirers, the unsolved question remained, whether non-constraint would be effective on a much larger scale in an asylum for many hundreds of inmates. The work of John Conolly MD was to show that it would. Early in his career, while practising at Stratford-upon-Avon, Conolly became an inspector of madhouses in the county; he published on the subject in 1830. Unable to make a successful livelihood in practice, in 1838 he was appointed as medical superintendent at Hanwell Asylum in Middlesex at £500 a year. His anti-restraint regime for four hundred inmates was at first sceptically received, but attracted the attention of *The Times* in the 1840s and came to be seen as a sign of Victorian humanity. In three years he had abolished all mechanical restraints and was employing more attendants instead. However, overcrowding became severe at Hanwell, with nearly a thousand patients in accommodation intended for only five hundred and a low cure rate. Although Hanwell trebled its bed capacity, it had failed to keep up with the expanding population of Middlesex and Colney Hatch Asylum was opened nearby in 1851 at a cost of nearly £300,000 in response to the problem. Conolly, stressing that 'every lunatic should be the property of the State', actively supported the building of county asylums, which some magistrates hoped to evade, and resigned when Middlesex tried to economise and to extend lay control at Hanwell. He published *The Construction and Government of Lunatic Asylums and Hospitals for the Insane* (1847) and *The Treatment of the Insane without Mechanical Restraints* (1856). Although elected FRCP for his work, he was savagely caricatured as Dr Wycherly in Charles Reade's novel, *Hard Cash* (1863). In spite of Conolly's reputation for non-coercion, he appears to have copied the regime from Lincoln Asylum, which he visited in 1838, run by Robert Gardiner Hill, who greatly resented his own lack of recognition and Conolly's later fame. Hill's ideas for asylum patients were too advanced for his own success, for he encouraged social contact between all classes of patients outside their own accommodation and abolished every kind of restraint for inmates. He was eventually forced to resign his appointment at the Lincoln Asylum.

The creation of some forty large-scale county lunatic asylums from the mid-nineteenth century was an unprecedented development in both psychiatric care and local government spending. Whereas under the Old Poor Law the expense of pauper lunatics was charged to the parish, the cost after 1834 was borne by the county, which actively encouraged parish officials to remove troublesome cases to a central institution. Also, under section 45 of the New Poor Law, lunatics were not to be kept in workhouses for longer than fourteen days and this too was an incentive for their removal. Later in the century, as overcrowding again became a problem, even larger asylums were built or older ones extended, so that some of the institutions were very expensive indeed, for example, £68,000 for Hatton, £114,831 for Arlesley. It is noticeable too that, as with eighteenth-century infirmaries, certain architects, such as G. T. Hine, G. F. Jones, H. E. Kendall and Scott & Moffatt, specialised in designing asylums, although they were not in the front rank of the profession. As with county infirmaries, competitions were held to build some asylums; thus at Coney Hill, Gloucester, where there were twenty-eight candidates, the contract was awarded to Giles and Gough, of Charing Cross, London. On such substantial contracts, for example, £80,000 to build Middlewood, Sheffield for eight hundred patients in 1872, the architect's 5 per cent fee was quite considerable. For virtually every asylum built, there were similar local difficulties, of funding, staffing and admission policies. Not all Poor Law unions were willing to contribute to the cost. The desperate need for accommodation, however, was common to all areas; thus in 1844 there were only forty places for lunatics in the North Riding of Yorkshire but 167 potential inmates.

Asylums soon began competing for inmates, undercutting rivals' charges and quoting bulk rates to the Poor Law unions to do so, and pauper lunatics would be moved from one asylum to another for cheaper terms. At Northampton the weekly rate was reduced from 10s. to 8s., while at Norfolk when 5s. 9½d. was charged for paupers, the non-poor paid 10s. a week. What could not have been predicted, however, was the considerable population growth after 1845, so that, by the end of the century, although the population had increased by 78 per cent, the numbers of insane had quadrupled and in 1890 comprised 30 in every ten thousand of the population. The huge increase, however, was noted in pauper rather than prosperous lunatics, and the 1830s and 1840s were the heyday of the large non-county pauper asylums, presumably in response to a market that could be profitably satisfied. These were especially noticeable in areas where counties were slow to build public institutions. Thus, in Herefordshire and Warwickshire three such establishments were opened in this period, holding 230 patients in all, where county asylums were not to be built until much later.

Various reasons have been suggested for this dramatic change in numbers. The data may have been unreliable, there could have been changed perceptions of what constituted madness, with society perhaps less tolerant towards bizarre, unacceptable behaviour, and it was widely agreed that the stresses of life were increasing. In addition, many occupations involved dangerous new techniques and substances. There also seems to have been a lower rate of cured patients, so that many were very long-term inmates, perhaps the longest a Norfolk woman in 1861 who had been a resident for sixty-six years. In the 1850s, the average length of stay in the York Lunatic Asylum was ten or eleven years. The best-known example of a long-stay patient in a county asylum was John Clare, the Northamptonshire lyrical poet, certified as suffering from 'hereditary madness'. He was treated for epileptiform fits as a youth and later in his life spent four years at Allen's private asylum in Epping Forest, his fees paid by friends. Becoming increasingly isolated and hallucinating, in December 1841 he was committed to the newly-built St Andrew's County Asylum at Northampton, where, however, he continued to write. He remained there until his death at the age of seventy, nearly twenty-three years later, his charge of 8s. a week paid by the local landowner, Earl Fitzwilliam. Modern diagnosis of his condition suggests that he suffered from cyclothymia (excessive mood swings).

By the 1840s the Lunacy Commissioners commented that it was increasingly difficult to find places for pauper lunatics and in 1856 they noted the 'crowded' county lunatic asylums and 'the urgent necessity' for more accommodation. County asylums had clearly become convenient places in which to incarcerate the difficult members of society. It is striking that the sheer size of the biggest made them the largest communities of the nineteenth century, far exceeding the size of factories, for example, so that Lancashire County Lunatic Asylum in 1848 had 750 inmates and in rural Northampton 850 patients could be accommodated. The Commissioners in Lunacy calculated that, whereas in 1850 there were twenty-four asylums with an average of 297 patients each, by 1870 there were an average of 549 patients in fifty-one institutions and, by 1870, these figures had risen to sixty-six asylums holding an average of 802 patients in each. County asylums continued to expand in size during the nineteenth century and many had two or three extensions added. After 1862 incurable but harmless pauper lunatics could be kept in their local workhouses, exactly as earlier in the century, consigning only the violent to the county asylum.

The new county asylums had certain features in common, apart from their architectural styles and semi-rural locations, with the Lunatic Commissioners requiring one acre for every four patients. The charge for keeping a patient there was twice the cost in a local workhouse and the age profile of inmates showed increasing numbers of elderly inmates, as at Hanwell, as life expectancy increased by the later nineteenth century. There had long been a stigma in being a county asylum patient and, in addition, before 1885 male pauper inmates were disenfranchised. The growth of the county asylum also produced new and experienced keepers as staff, who could make a career as more institutions were built and expanded. However, the ratio of staff to inmates remained an acute problem, especially when comparisons were made between the county asylum and the privately-run establishment. Thus at Newcastle upon Tyne Lunatic Asylum in 1827 eighty inmates, almost all paupers, had nine attendants, while at the town's private establishment at the same period seventeen inmates were also cared for by nine staff. Similarly, at Ticehurst there was one attendant for every two patients, while in even the better county asylum, with over a thousand patients, the ratio was 1: 10 or 1: 12, clearly reflected in the charges to inmates (in 1879), £470 a year for an inmate at Ticehurst in contrast to about £100 a year in the public institution. Activities for patients were obviously determined by the numbers of staff to supervise them, but at Mrs Bradbury's establishment near London for wealthy 'ladies nervously affected' a coloured print of about 1830 shows ten inmates in the garden, chatting, walking, skipping and playing the guitar.

Occasionally, a lunacy case would receive very wide publicity, usually because of the status of those involved, and in the 1870s the most striking example of this phenomenon was the melodrama involving Lady Mordaunt and the Prince of Wales. Not only was it a lurid tale of adultery in high places, but its outcome, the incarceration of Lady Mordaunt as a lunatic, became an important legal and medical precedent in cases of puerperal insanity. In 1866 the beautiful Harriett Moncrieffe, at eighteen, had married Sir Charles Mordaunt of Walton, 10th Baronet, a Warwickshire MP. In London's fashionable circles, Edward, Prince of Wales was quickly attracted to her, as were a number of others in the royal set, but Sir Charles's suspicions of her behaviour were confirmed when he discovered that Edward regularly visited Lady Mordaunt, unaccompanied, both in London and in the country. When her first child was born in 1869, Lady Mordaunt confessed that Sir Charles was not the father and that the infant's eye infection was the result of a venereal condition caught from one of her lovers. Edward, Lord Cole was the chief suspect. When Sir Charles demanded a divorce on the grounds of adultery, Lady Mordaunt showed symptoms of madness and a divorce could not then be granted against a person of unsound mind. In 1875, as the result of a change in the divorce laws, Sir Charles gained his freedom because of Harriett's adultery with Lord Cole. Lady Mordaunt remained in various private mental institutions for some thirty years until her death in 1906. The Mordaunt case, however, was of considerable medical significance and featured at length in *The Medical Times and Gazette* of 1870, in an article which discussed Lady

Mordaunt's symptoms of puerperal mania in a melancholic form. The dozen medical experts used by both Sir Charles and the Moncrieffe family were the acknowledged leaders in the field, including Sir James Simpson, Sir James Alderson, Dr Harrington Tuke, Dr Forbes Winslow and Dr William Priestley. *The Medical Times* considered that this 'grave public scandal' rested on a failure to distinguish the condition of puerperal melancholia from that of puerperal mania and should have been settled in private.

Towards the end of the nineteenth century fears were growing about wrongful detention in asylums and in 1890 the Lunacy Act (53 Vict. c. 5) was passed to curb this abuse, requiring a magistrate's order for a patient's admission. The fact that a JP could override medical opinion about a patient's admission, and also that the Act contained three hundred and forty two clauses, caused considerable medical resentment and the Act was described by a contemporary as 'cumbersome and difficult to work', not least because of the amout of form-filling it required. In addition, a certificate was required before mechanical restraint could be used and the amount of extra work for medical superintendents in asylums necessitated the appointment of a second medical officer at Bethlem, for example. However, one of the main results of the Act was a fall in the numbers of certified patients and a rise in voluntary admissions in the period 1900–16 as the stigma attached to certification was removed.

Forty years later the Mental Treatment Act of 1930 replaced the phrase 'lunatic asylum' by 'mental hospital' and extended the principle of voluntary admissions to all hospitals. There was a noticeable growth in out-patient treatment, although Bethlem had opened the first London psychiatric outpatient department before the 1930 Act. These departments grew rapidly and their numbers rose from only 25 in 1930 to 162 by 1935. However, even in 1938 there were still thirty-one private asylums in the provinces. The 1959 Mental Health Act reflected the growing interest in community-based mental care and the Act allowed psychiatric patients to be treated in general hospitals as part of the NHS. Some compulsory detention still existed, but patients were allowed the right of appeal.

Huge changes in psychiatric medicine have been seen in the last decades of the twentieth century as care in the community has replaced detention in a mental hospital. A government decision has meant that, of the 121 asylums operational in 1986, 98 were to close by the year 2000. Some of the grandest asylum buildings themselves have become derelict and vandalised, for example, Exe Vale Hospital, others demolished to make way for a new housing estate (Hatton). Some asylums have seen the building of modern houses in the grounds, as at Bracebridge Heath and Lincoln and some main hospital buildings have themselves been converted into flats (Colney Hatch, Haywards Heath). Institutional uses are also possible, as at Cranage Hall, now a conference centre. Only a handful, such as St Andrews, Northampton, continue in their original role as asylums.

Prisons

From the earliest times, all English counties and many towns had gaols and bridewells where felons and debtors could be imprisoned; even smaller communities had a lock-up, as at Ripon (1686). These gaols were often, until the later eighteenth century, very ancient buildings and John Howard (1726?–1790), the Dissenter, noted those at Chesterfield (founded in 1614), Halifax (1670) Hertford (1702) and Shrewsbury (1705) still functioning as prisons at the time of his visit in the late 1770s. All were exceptionally overcrowded and insanitary, while the conditions at Oxford reminded him of one of the city's great gaol epidemics, the Black Assize, in the past. However, all gaols regularly experienced outbreaks of fevers and other infections, their inmates living closely confined, badly lodged and fed, often the poorest members of society. There is no distinct period when gaol surgeons began to be appointed, although they appear regularly in Quarter Sessions papers by the seventeenth century, paid for providing medicines and treatment to prisoners, and arranging inquests when necessary. The gaol surgeon usually lived near the prison and his appointment was part-time. Such duties were not arduous for the small numbers of criminals in pre-industrial England, but expanded along with the population by the later eighteenth century and were greatly increased when, as a result of war, convicts could no longer be transported to the American colonies after 1775 and the prison population swelled. The numbers of inmates noted by John Howard indicate that a serious health problem was imminent and public interest was aroused, either for philanthropic reasons or through personal fears of infection.

In 1773–6, 1779 and 1782 Howard travelled nearly 25,000 miles and inspected every English prison two or three times, as well as five tours in Europe, demanding improved sanitary conditions for the inmates and noting 'close and offensive' conditions virtually everywhere. In 1774 an Act was passed (14 Geo. III, c. 59) intended to protect prisoners' health, by limewashing gaol walls and providing separate sickrooms. The first edition of Howard's *The State of the Prisons in England and Wales* appeared three years later. He commented that smallpox was commonplace and that some prison officials had died in outbreaks of gaol fever (typhus), including the gaoler at Warwick and the turnkey at Chelmsford. At Bedford the surgeon had died in an epidemic, while at Exeter the surgeon's contract specifically excluded his attendance at typhus cases. The Worcester prison surgeon, John Hallward, 'caught the gaol-fever some years ago, and ever since has been fearful of going into the dungeon: when any felon is sick there, he orders him to be brought out'. Unhappily, the young physician, Edward Johnstone, newly appointed to the county hospital there, decided to attend typhus victims in the castle gaol and died himself from the infection. That prisoners were acknowledged as a risk to the public can be seen in the Hertfordshire Quarter Sessions accounts in 1774, when £1 19s. was spent on new clothes for prisoners 'to make them clean and free from infection for their Trials'. Not surprisingly, Howard was often asked how he avoided infection, especially typhus, in his prison visits; his response was:

Next to the free goodness and mercy of the Author of my being, tem-
perance and cleanliness are my chief preservatives ... I visit the most
infectious hospitals and noxious cells; and while thus employed, I fear
no evil. However, I seldom enter a hospital or prison before breakfast;
in an offensive room I avoid drawing my breath deeply; and on my
return sometimes wash my mouth and hands.

He was pleased to record when new prisons were built, as at Ely (1768),
Manchester (1774) and Liverpool (1776), but even at Coventry, where the gaol
was only two years old, Howard described conditions as 'dirty, offensive and
unhealthy ... no infirmary'. Howard had scientific Quaker support in his
demands for prison reforms, which included uniforms, baths, delousing, a regular
diet and medical inspections of prisoners, for whom he believed strict and unwelcome hygienic conditions would bring moral improvement and discipline. He
noted fewer than ten institutions with infirmaries for sick prisoners. As a result
of his efforts, a competition was arranged for plans to erect prisons under the
Penitentiary Act of 1779 and, although these were never built, the prize-winning
architect was William Blackburn (1750–90). This success brought him commissions to design a total of eighteen prisons, bridewells and houses of correction,
including county gaols for Devon, Oxfordshire and Suffolk. Perhaps surprisingly,
several eminent architects, such as John Carr, John Nash and Sir John Soane,
also designed prisons, and the years up to about 1825 saw a number of very large
purpose-built gaols erected across the country and a further remarkable growth
in the 1840s and 1850s.

A leading influence in prison reform was Sir George Onesiphorous Paul
(1746–1820), who pressed for change after a disastrous outbreak of typhus in
Gloucester Castle (then the county gaol) when it was seriously overcrowded in
1784. Paul had to convince his fellow magistrates that a hygienic ritual would be
additional punishment to the inmates, and shaved prisoners' heads as a further
deterrent. He insisted that there was 'a moral as well as a physical purpose to be
served' in Gloucester prison, where a regular diet was provided and only two
family visits a year were permitted to inmates, who were not allowed bedding, furniture or books. A new county gaol and five houses of correction to hold between
four and five hundred prisoners were built there in 1792 at a cost to the county of
£46,000. Following an outbreak of gaol fever in 1783, a number of counties on the
Oxford circuit began erecting new purpose-built gaols. Hereford was one of these,
where a new gaol was built in the years 1792–7 at a cost of £18,646 16s. 3¼d. It
was a commission John Nash carried out fairly early in his professional career,
having already designed similar gaols for two Welsh counties and at a time when
he was also engaged on two other country house projects in Herefordshire.
Although the governor's house survived, the gaol was demolished in 1930.

These institutions all needed the services of a medical practitioner, and this
was a category of professional work that expanded considerably from the
mid-eighteenth century. Many gaol surgeons' case-books, especially from the

nineteenth century, have survived to illustrate their activities, for which contracts were usually arranged. Prisons, in fact, were, with workhouses, the earliest public institutions to offer medical service contract appointments. In the eighteenth century such part-time posts added to a practitioner's total income, with guaranteed prompt payments and patients that were presumably less demanding than those usually attended for individual fees. John Howard noted whether prison surgeons received 'salaries' (virtually a contract fee) or submitted bills for their attention, but charges were always low, a salary of £20 at Warwick, for example, while the chaplain there had £50 a year. Other annual fees Howard recorded included £5 5s. at Horsham, £10 10s. at Marlborough and £25 at Oxford for attending the felons, of whom there were 31 in 1782. Even at Newgate in the same year, with 291 felons, the surgeon's salary was only £100. The influence of Howard's inspections can be clearly seen in the building programmes that six counties undertook after he had publicly condemned their existing prisons. Thus York, where he saw only fourteen inmates in 1779, rebuilt its prison at considerable expense in 1802–7 to the design of Peter Atkinson junior, the first public commission of this local architect. The prison, demolished in 1880, had a bath room and regularly employed a surgeon before required to do so by law. As well as treating prisoners that were obviously sick, the surgeon also inspected the buildings to judge standards of hygiene, heard inmates' complaints (often about their diet) and certified prisoners fit for transportation. The surgeon could also advise on the level of work prisoners might perform (whether fit enough for the treadmill), if alcohol could be recommended or a sick prisoner's shackles removed.

In spite of Howard's efforts and those of his successor, James Neild (1744–1814), the zeal for prison reform was fading by the early years of the nineteenth century, perhaps to concentrate on factory and labour abuses, but the concept of work for prisoners and a hygienic ritual were not to survive, as illustrated in the riots at Coldbath Fields prison, where inmates complained to the Middlesex magistrates of cold, damp, inadequate rations and 'swarms of mice rattling in their rooms'. Solitary confinement was attacked as repressive, but the general prison population swelled when it was discontinued. Epidemics were particularly virulent for inmates fed on only bread and water, although the increased use of whitewashing, baths and uniforms was to prevent a high death rate in Newgate's dangerously overcrowded years (1815–19), and its last serious epidemic had occurred in 1802–3, when seventy-nine prisoners died.

Suspicions that prisoners were being too well treated led to a reduction in rations, loss of privileges (no reading material, silent exercise and fewer family visits) and at Millbank food was reduced so much that in the winter of 1823 there were four hundred ill from outbreaks of typhus, scurvy and dysentery, with thirty-one deaths. The prison was closed until 1824 and the inmates released or sent elsewhere. The coroner's jury were persuaded to pronounce a verdict of accidental deaths, although they initially blamed 'inadequate diet'.

The coming of the Pentonville system in 1842 and the general professionalisation of the whole prison service meant that medical personnel would have an integral role in the prisons, and certainly by the mid-nineteenth century regular, often daily, medical attendance was provided at all gaols. However, even a new prison building could not necessarily avoid brutality to prisoners and illegal punishments as a means of control. Thus Birmingham's new prison at Winson Green, opened in 1849 with cells for 321 inmates, witnessed a great scandal only four years later when, overcrowded, prisoners were punished by deprivation of diet, excessive use of the crank and a straitjacket as a means of physical control. Criminal charges were brought against both the governor, who was sent to prison, and the surgeon. The level of health care in prisons predictably improved in step with general improvements in medical attention to the population at large and by 1877 the modern penal system was in place. Nearly half of the actual Victorian buildings were still in use in 1969.

A visit to Nottingham Asylum, 1814

We arrived at Nottingham at 5 to dinner ... After dinner about ½p. 6 a note to Dr. Pennington requesting permission to see the Asylum. The Dr. immediately called upon us, and took us thither. It is a new building, and stands delightfully on the slope of a hill, about ½ a mile from the centre of the town; without side suburbs. It has only been finished about 2 years; & is on a most excellent plan.

Tho' we took them by surprise we found eveything clean & orderly. There are 54 patients. The building would hold 84. This Asylum is on a mixed plan of constitution, being partly built at the expense of the County as a place for Parish paupers, & partly by subscription for other Lunatics.

Except in one or two instances of double bedded rooms, every patient has a distinct lodging room; & the provisions for air & ventilation are excellent; there are six spacious airing courts for the patients to walk in; & a large garden.

We introduced ourselves to Dr. P. as Governors of the York Asylum; which it appears was not the most flattering mode we cd. have adopted; tho' the Doctor's civility was equal to what it would have been under the most favourable circumstances of introduction ...

This certainly is a place where any person might send their friends with satisfaction. The rooms for the opulent patients are handsomely furnished; & they are allowed their own servants if they wish it. Those for the poor are very airy, clean & comfortable. The bare mention of our mode of proceeding at York makes them stare with astonishment. The building &c. cost 20,000£ ...

Dr. P. rec^s 1 gns. per ann. for paupers besides 9s p. week which is paid to the institution: 2 gns. p. ann. from patients who pay less than 1 gna. a week to the Inst^n 4 gns. p. ann. from those who pay 1 gna. 6 gns. from those who are charged 1 gna. & a half; & 8 gns. p. ann. from those who pay 2 gns. or

upwards p. week. Patients may be charged 3 gns. or more p. week according to their circumstances. There is an excellent Apothecary & Matron.

Mrs Edwin Gray, *Papers and Diaries of a York family*, 1927, pp. 134–5

The Gloucester City gaol surgeon's journal, 1827 and 1828

1827
23 September Wight cured of the Itch & all the transports are fit for
removal. No complaint to the Prison.
24 September Examined the transports & certified they were all fit for
removal. No complaint.
1 November Visited the different department of the prison. No complaint.
26 December Prisoners are in perfect Health.

1828
3 February Visited: Frith a boy who is subject to fits should not work on the
Wheel at least not at those time when he may be expected to have them,
they are periodical being influenced by the particular State of the Moon
have given him Medicines the others are well.
22 March Two Felons are complaining – both Venereal disease & one has
also the Itch. An old Man named White complains of Asthma – he should
have but light work on the Wheel – Several convicted Prisoners complained of their Bread being short weight. I find on enquiry this is true &
that Mr Turner has frequently return'd the loaves and got them changed.
3 April Visited
15 April Edwards has an inflamed Eye from cold, sent him an application
for it. The others are tolerable.
16 April Charlotte Smith and Ann Clutterbuck are both Itch'd
21 April Visited the Prison
22 April Visited
29 April Visited the Prison
2 May Visited Browning is much debilitated by a Venereal disease he has
been affected with & appears too much reduced to be able to work much
at the Wheel – I advise his being allowed ½ a pint of Porter daily.
6 May Visited the Prisoners generally. Browning is better.
23 May Browning is quite well and may discontinue the Porter, and pursue
the labour of the Tread Mill with the other Prisoners.
12 July Visited the Prison
22 August Visited the Prison
28 August Nicholas Salter has a venereal complaint which however is not
a sufficient excuse for his not working on the Wheel.

Gloucestershire Record Office, QBR/G3/G8/1

There are two men's initials at the end of these comments; the practitioners appear to be Messrs Washbourne, apothecaries and druggists in East Street, Gloucester.

MIDWIFERY AND NURSING

Dr Ford ... has been with me this morning & he almost certainly confirms my
suspicions that my child has been dead some time. He won't say that he is certain
of it but that it is *most* probable. But he assures me I shall continue very well
until the time & then he says I shall be in no more danger than if the child were
alive & shall recover afterwards faster than usual. ... I hope with a proper trust in
God I shall be able to go on through this affair.

Malcolm Elwin, *The Noels and the Milbankes*, 1967, p. 185

Unhappily, this distressed patient wrote to her aunt in November 1781 but was
dead, at the age of twenty-four, in the following year. However, her case illustrates that, even for the wealthy lady with a senior London practitioner in attendance, childbirth was a hazardous and often life-threatening experience. Since
reliable contraception simply did not exist before the twentieth century, most
married women spent at least two decades of their lives either pregnant or fearing
that they were so. Medical attention in pregnancy, as in other conditions, varied
according to the patient's prosperity and ranged from the society *accoucheur* to
Sairey Gamp. Although in England male midwives were not common until the
1750s, practitioners with special skills, such as Percival Willoughby, existed a
century earlier.

Even by the early eighteenth century the church was legally responsible for
licensing a female midwife to practise. To obtain a bishop's licence she was
required to be a woman of good character, vouched for by local worthies
and women she had attended; she also had to be able to pay the licence fee.
This was often more than a poorer applicant could afford, and in *Tristram
Shandy* in the 1760s the parson paid Mrs Wood's fee of 18s. 4d. to enable her
to obtain a licence to practise. The midwife was to christen the child if it were
likely to die, prevent substitution of a live baby for a dead one and, if the infant
were stillborn, witness that the mother had not killed the child. If the
birth were illegitimate, the midwife was also to persuade the mother to name
the child's father, thereby passing on the costs of paternity from the poor rate.
She took an oath that she would help poor women in labour as well as rich, not
use

witchcraft, not induce an abortion and not deliver a child in secret. Furthermore: If any child be dead-born (she was to) see it buried in such secret place as neither hog nor dog nor any other beast may come unto it [nor] suffer any such child to be cast into the jacques [latrine] or any other inconvenient place

Midwives' moral standing was frequently suspect; thus Mrs Mandrake in George Farquhar's *The Twin Rivals* (1702) was a midwife/procuress and their presumed knowledge of how to effect an abortion made them particularly suspect, as represented by Defoe's Mother Midnight in *Moll Flanders* (1722). They have always been traditionally associated with witchcraft, especially practices involving the use of the placenta. Their reputation for drinking was at least Elizabethan in origin, and 'like aqua vitae with a midwife' must have been a widely-popular enough phrase to be thought amusing in *Twelfth Night*. The Rowlandson cartoon (Figure 7.1) and Sairey Gamp kept the unflattering image alive for two centuries.

However, most midwives were of humble status, ill-educated, with modest fees and a professional standing well below that of their male rivals. They were often widows, since it was thought unsuitable for spinsters to be involved in childbirth, and their patients ranged from the pauper to the aristocrat, with fees adjusted accordingly. There were no requirements for their education and training, although many midwives were trained by their mothers and a few were apprenticed to an experienced woman. Percival Willoughby's own daughter assisted him as a midwife in London and Staffordshire, and was presumably trained by her father, who had, in his *Observations in Midwifery*, some extreme criticisms of incompetent midwives, whose interventions often killed the patient. Generally midwives have been described as completely illiterate, although their manuscripts occasionally survive to suggest otherwise. A remarkable example was the casebook kept by an anonymous London midwife for the years 1694–1723, ill-written but recording the 687 deliveries she attended, an average of just over twenty-four a year. Her fees ranged from 2s. 6d. to £1 16s., but with 10s. most often recorded and in 1704 she earned the highest sum, £50 2s. 8d., from thirty-seven cases. There were a striking number of patients she attended for six or more pregnancies and they included the wives of craftsmen, traders and gentry. She travelled to some thirty parishes in London, and although most of her patients lived in the Chancery Lane and Old Bailey areas, she also went as far as Leytonstone in Essex. Unfortunately she has, however, never been identified.

It is clear that midwives' skills must invariably have been acquired from observation and experience rather than books, for there were no texts in English they could use until the publication of Jane Sharp's *The Midwives Book* (1671) and, in the same year, William Sermon's *The Ladies Companion or the English Midwife*. As a midwife herself, Jane Sharp condemned her male rivals, adding that poor country people, assisted only by women 'are as fruitful, and as safe and well delivered, if not much more fruitful and better commonly in childbed than the

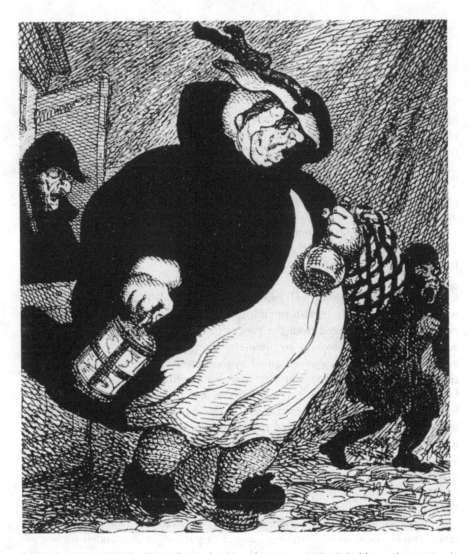

Figure 7.1 A cartoon by Thomas Rowlandson showing a midwife holding a lantern and bottle of spirits, 1811.

greatest Ladies of the Land'. There was general consensus that a midwife's task was to deliver a live child, while a male practitioner was sought in a crisis to deliver a dead one. *Accoucheurs'* and midwives' views of childbirth differed in the most significant aspects; thus, a male practitioner would have the newly-delivered woman lie in a prone position for three or four days after giving birth, reasonably to prevent the prolapsed uterus so common after a woman had endured many pregnancies. The midwife and her local female helpers, however, always advised that the patient should be out of bed and walking around twenty-four hours after delivery to remove lochial discharge, a view later widely accepted.

It was not until half a century later that Sarah Stone published her *Complete Practice of Midwifery* (1737), claiming that she had practised for thirty-five years, having worked under her mother for six; she thought three years training was essential. She was opposed to midwives using instruments to assist delivery, although Chamberlen's obstetric forceps had been available since 1728. She claimed to have delivered over three hundred women a year in the Taunton area. Although a midwife's workload is difficult to estimate, if only for lack of sources, one woman's obituary notice in 1767 said that she had delivered ten thousand patients in forty-five years, some four a week. A midwife's value to her community must have been considerable, echoed in one woman's epitaph, which Lord Torrington noted in 1781: she was 'compassionate to the afflicted, kind to her relations, and very skilful in midwifery'. Since there was no register of midwives at this period, it is impossible to discover how many women were actually practising their skills. The trade directories for the eighteenth century include only the occasional midwives, certainly not enough to deliver all the women lying in. At Worcester in 1794, for example, a directory named only one midwife, clearly not able to provide for a city's needs, while at Hereford none was listed. In Warwick, while only one midwife was noted in the official trade directory, other sources, especially poor law records, suggest there were another four midwives regularly practising in the town. However, *The Universal British Directory* of the mid-1790s erratically noted midwives in some large northern towns, including Manchester (4) and Newcastle upon Tyne (7). To indicate the availability of the *accoucheur*, the same publication listed 265 provincial surgeon-apothecaries who were also men-midwives, as obstetric work increasingly became an important part of a practitioner's income, especially for the prosperous patient. Robert Smith, an eighteenth-century Bristol surgeon, held the view that for a practitioner, midwifery work could not be adequately rewarded by the 'mere lying in fee, unless it leads to other business' and responsibility for the general health of a family.

Undoubtedly the early decades of the eighteenth century saw the rise of the man-midwife in Britain at the same time that episcopal licensing of women was declining, as in London by the 1720s. In most provincial dioceses licences cannot be found after this period, although at Peterborough a midwife's licence was granted as late as 1818 and at Lichfield in 1821. At the same time that changes were taking place in midwifery practice and practitioners, there were also the beginnings of institutional care in pregnancy. As early as 1739 Sir Richard Manningham, a leading London *accoucheur*, made available two wards in St James's Infirmary, Westminster, for married women to give birth and where he took both male and female pupils in midwifery. William Cadogan MD commented in his *Essay Upon Nursing* (1748) that 'it is with great Pleasure that I see at last the Preservation of Children become the Care of the Men of Sense', his fellow practitioners. Lying-in facilities were provided at the Middlesex (1747), the British (1749), the City of London (1750), Queen Charlotte's and the Westminster hospitals, mainly, under a moral exclusion rule, as charities for married women, although the last two, both founded in 1752, would admit spinsters, but only for a first birth. Provincial lying-in facilities were virtually non-existent, although at Bristol a charity was founded in 1777 to deliver poor married women in their own homes, attended by two men-midwives. Nearly all lying-in hospitals excluded first births to married women and also those who had no child living, as well as those with disabled or diseased children. It was not until the later nineteenth century, 1899 in Liverpool, for example, that most charities would accept the unmarried mother, and then only if respectable and not 'of profligate status', although at the time there were some two hundred single women a year giving birth in the city's workhouses.

Such charitable provisions for poor women were extremely rare at this period. The Revd David Davies recorded in 1795 that poor families needed to allocate £1 once in two years for the expenses of childbirth, made up of 3s. or 4s. for the child's linen, 5s. for the midwife's fee (a sum widely charged), a bottle of brandy or gin 'always had upon this occasion' at 2s., half a bushel of malt and hops at 3s., a nurse for a few days, including her diet, cost at least 5s. and, finally, a shilling to the incumbent for the churching ceremony. The total charge to the parish of a birth, however, could be as much as £5, but the midwife attended only a minority of all pauper births. Midwives certainly did not live in every small village and entries in Overseers' accounts for fetching the midwife are commonplace, with horse hire if necessary. By the early nineteenth century town parishes with large numbers of pauper births transformed the midwifery fees into an annual contract sum, such as £3 at Stratford-upon-Avon in 1813, for example. Midwives could also be asked to examine ('search') those claiming to be pregnant and they would also treat women for mastitis ('a bad breast') and reduce the level of lactation by 'drawing' a patient's breasts. A midwife's clientèle could extend from paupers to ladies, although the fees differed considerably, and in some grand families a successful delivery would bring the midwife a gift of several guineas.

The midwifery picture in London was completely different from that in the provinces. In the capital there were some fifteen physicians who were also noted as men-midwives in the 1783 *Medical Register*, famous consultants such as Thomas Denman and William Bromfield, who had extensive private practices as well as their posts at the lying-in hospitals. The status of midwifery was undoubtedly enhanced by the work of William Smellie and William Hunter, both Scots, who delivered great ladies for substantial fees and thus became nationally known, especially as pregnancy increasingly came to be seen as an illness and midwifery accordingly medicalised. However, in the provinces obstetric work was carried out by the surgeon-apothecaries, typified by Thomas W. Jones of Henley-in-Arden, who kept careful casenotes of the women he delivered during a decade. Of his 422 cases (one every five or six days) he noted fees and delivery details. His usual charge was 10s. 6d., although more for a protracted labour or for the local gentry, and he covered an area within a five-mile radius of his surgery. He too was less than pleased at the efforts of local female midwives, noting for one patient that he 'delivered with great difficulty on account of the Hand being so exceedingly low down. Mrs Doley had attended – the Child Dead'. Mrs Elizabeth Doley also worked as poor law midwife to three parishes nearby. Such rivalry was inevitable and a century earlier Percival Willoughby had expressed his anger when he was called to protracted deliveries at which the local midwife's efforts had proved in vain, often with fatal results for the patient. However, medical views diverged on the subject, for in 1773 Dr Charles White, a well-known man-midwife, in his *Treatise on the Management of Pregnant and Lying-in Women*, could comment that the death-rate of poor women, delivered only by an ignorant local midwife, might be lower than patients in lying-in hospitals or the affluent ladies delivered by the *accoucheur*, both groups equally at risk from fatal puerperal fever by cross-infection, a danger also recognised by Alexander Gordon at the same period.

Clearly, respectable village midwives suffered a loss of patients, status and income once male practitioners were widely accepted as superior, and the picture of Leah Cousins superseded by Dr Glibb that George Crabbe gave in his *Parish Register* of 1807 must have been typical. As male obstetricians became more popular, many practitioners saw such work as a means of practice-expansion, very necessary in the increasingly competitive business of nineteenth-century medicine. A degree of patient-loyalty can be seen in midwifery work, as most women experienced many pregnancies in their lives and regularly employed the same *accoucheur* or midwife on each occasion. There were, however, popular moral objections raised against male midwives in Georgian England; it was claimed that they seduced patients and that female virtue had declined, although French novels and dances, as well as boarding schools, were also blamed for this phenomenon.

In spite of some famous practitioners undertaking and charging large fees for midwifery work, it was generally held in low esteem by the profession. There were no special qualifications, but some eminent practitioners lectured privately in London. In 1841 the Royal College of Surgeons had a separate midwifery examination and three years later offered a diploma in midwifery; the subject was already compulsory at Edinburgh University and on the continent. The Apothecaries' Act (1815) did not initially require licentiates to hold a midwifery qualification, although it was later added, and the Medical Act of 1886 required a midwifery qualification for those listed in the *Medical Register*. The Royal College of Physicians still resisted, however, considering that, as a manual operation, it was 'foreign to the habits of Gentlemen of enlarged academical education' to practise obstetrics, a view presented to the 1834 Select Committee on Medical Education.

In the nineteenth century the influence of Florence Nightingale was to be felt in the whole area of midwife training. By this period there were surplus women, not all of working class status, seeking employment and more work was available for midwives in a population boom. However, midwives possessed none of the

125

symbols of a profession – they had no publication or register of members and their training opportunities were negligible. Educated, respectable women would have been deterred from an occupation whose best-known figure was the fictional Sairey Gamp. Even royal babies were not safe from the attentions of a drunken midwife, as a cartoon of 1842 vividly illustrated, showing the infant Prince of Wales being given alcohol by his midwife. Lord Shaftesbury was president of the Female Medical Society, founded in 1863, with one of its objects the training of gentlewomen as midwives, but it survived for only ten years. Florence Nightingale rightly considered that better midwifery services would be provided for all if local women could be centrally trained and then return to their own areas. She thus set up an innovative training scheme in which village women, sponsored by their parishioners, were trained as midwives in London for six months and then went home to aid the rural poor. Unfortunately, the scheme lasted only seven years, for she had not considered the domestic difficulties for the trainees when they had young children of their own, who had to be cared for in their mother's absence. However, in the later nineteenth century female education was improving, enabling women to undertake more careers than the traditional role of governess, and midwifery gradually became an acceptable occupation as it grew towards professionalism. The Midwives' Act of 1902 required certification and in 1905 a Select Committee pronounced in favour of a midwives' register, with a central body, state-run, to approve training schools and admit qualified candidates, with experience and a good character, to the register.

A specialised area of nursing, available to only the affluent, was that of the monthly nurse, caring for the mother and baby and assisting the *accoucheur*, delivering the baby if necessary. She was to arrive in the house before the birth and, from the evidence of eighteenth-century gentry correspondence, there was considerable competition to secure the services of certain women. Some monthly nurses had a remarkable clientèle amongst the aristocracy and fashion seems often to have dictated a lady's choice, as in selecting her obstetrician. Training for monthly nurses was arranged at the British Lying-In Hospital in 1826 and at Queen Charlotte's Hospital in 1851.

Nursing

Florence Nightingale considered nursing an art and a vocation, requiring:

> As exclusive a devotion, as hard a preparation, as any painter's or sculptor's work; for what is the having to do with dead canvas or cold marble compared with having to do with the living body – the temple of God's spirit. It is one of the Arts; I had almost said, the finest of the Fine Arts.

Her *Notes on Nursing*, published in 1860, sold 15,000 copies in the first two months and continued to be reprinted until the end of the nineteenth century. Much slower to attain respectability and professional status than midwifery, nursing was generally considered to be the responsibility of a patient's family and the Poor Law authorities were reluctant to provide the most basic nursing attention if the family could do so. Women referred to as nurses, for all patients, were untrained, except by experience, and really carried out orderly duties, providing essential attendance for the bedridden. Charges for nursing or attendance are among the commonest of all payments in Old Poor Law accounts, providing not only assistance to the patient but also small cash sums to other parishioners for carrying out the essential duties. The nurse might also lay out the former patient and clean and dress the corpse ready for burial, but this, the most menial of tasks, was generally performed for pennies by old village women of even lower status than the nurse. Nursing attention after childbirth usually lasted for a month. The rate of pay for parish nursing was 2s. a week in the period 1750–75, increasing by the 1790s to 3s.6d. and to 4s. by the early nineteenth century. Further small payments were made to nurses who sat up at night with a patient. The parish nurse's duties consisted of making the patient comfortable, doing laundry and preparing food, as well as often looking after the children and husband of a sick woman. However, some poor law nurses were clearly more skilled and undertook a wider range of duties; one woman at Farnborough in the early 1790s was paid for attending a sore leg and dressing various limbs, for which she received shillings, not pence.

A clear but narrow picture of nursing in the eighteenth and nineteenth centuries, however, comes from institutions, the voluntary infirmaries and the workhouse hospitals, whose staff were described and criticised by many commentators. In the years 1736–97 a total of twenty-eight hospitals opened in the English provinces, some of considerable size, all with distinguished physicians and surgeons as their honorary staff (see Chapter 5), but with apparently no thought having been given to skilled nursing assistance. It is also, however, clear that infirmary governors were more concerned with the honesty and sobriety of their matron and nursing staff than any professional skills, for drunkenness and theft were the most commonly recorded complaints against hospital staff throughout the eighteenth and early nineteenth centuries. The matron's duties were primarily those of a housekeeper; she was responsible for the domestic bills, as well as controlling the nursing staff, porters and other hospital servants. For Worcester Infirmary, where she was paid £6 a year, plus a gratuity, the post was advertised in 1778 in two county newspapers. In his travels, John Howard commented that 'with respect to health and convenience in workhouses and infirmaries, more depends on such women [matrons] than is generally imagined'. At this period, Worcester always had two or three nurses but the whole wage bill there was never more than 10 per cent of the total running charges. Nurses there were paid £3 10s. a year plus a gratuity and in 1774 they asked the Governors for either more nurses to be employed or to have a pay rise; their wage was increased to £6 a year. These posts were residential and the women were given free board, lodging and washing. At Winchester, where the matron received the larger wage of £15 15s. a year, the five nurses had only £2 10s. each. At St Thomas's Hospital in London, with some five hundred patients, the matron was paid the large annual wage of £60. Sisters, who had often been head servants in large households, earned £30 or £40 a year. At the London Hospital, soon after its opening in 1740, nurses were paid £6 a year and their duties were clearly defined:

> To enter upon their Business every morning at six in Summer, and at seven in Winter, to sup at ten and be in bed by eleven every Night; to clean their wards, pewter and utensils every day by seven in the morning; to attend the patients diligently during their Watch, and provide them with what is directed by the Physician, Surgeon and Apothecary, and see particularly that they take their medicines, and to keep the beds of the Patients neat and decent.

They were also required to 'behave with Tenderness to the Patients and with Curtesy and Respect to Strangers'.

At Northampton, where there were three nurses and a porter for thirty beds in the mid-eighteenth century, nurses were paid £5 a year and £2 gratuity, while the matron had £10 a year. The hospital expanded considerably by 1793, with 90 to 100 beds, for which there were four nurses and three maids. By 1805 the Governors decided that a matron at Northampton should be aged between thirty and forty-five, but she was to be paid £21 a year plus £4 12s. in lieu of her ale and tea allowances. The longevity of some hospital nurses was remarkable; at Northampton there was one aged seventy-five in 1806 and in 1845 one of eighty. These women and several others of great age received small annuities from the Governors. The longest-serving matron there for thirty years, retiring in 1794, was Mrs Mary Knapton, who was given an obituary notice in the *Gentleman's Magazine* in 1805:

> At Whiston, co. Northampton, in her 91st year, Mrs Knapton, 30 years matron of the County Infirmary; and as a reward for the fidelity with which she executed that trust, the Governors, when age obliged her to resign the situation, settled upon her £20 a year for the rest of her life.

She had obviously retired at the age of eighty; her annual salary had been £20.

It was not until the mid-nineteenth century, however, that night nurses were employed; before this, night care had been in the hands of casual women from the town. In 1866 when Northampton advertised for assistant nurses at £10 a year they were required to be able to read and write. By the 1870s nurses were being admitted to the hospital for training. An interesting picture of life at Northampton was given in a letter to Florence Nightingale in 1889 from Margaret Winterton, the newly-appointed superintendent of nurses:

> The wards are nice, but we are terribly undernursed – each head nurse has charge of thirty patients, divided into four wards with only one assistant day nurse and a night nurse, and they have not only all the

patients to tend, meals to serve, etc., but all the floors to sweep and polish with beeswax every week, windows to clean and, in fact, charwomen's work to do. The nurses take alternately *one week* day duty and *one week* night duty, so that it is perpetual change, and every other Sunday when they change from day to night duty they are on duty from 6.30 a.m. till 7 p.m., when they are supposed to go to bed till 9.30 p.m. (2 ½ hours) and then go on duty again all night and not to bed till after the ordinary mid-day dinner at 1 p.m. on Monday ...There are no meals prepared for the nurses, they have to get and clear away their own, and altogether it seems such a heathenish place that I do not feel I can settle or do any good here.

The dissatisfied Miss Winterton stayed for only three years. However, at Northampton, as in other hospitals, conditions were improving for nurses and by 1901 a nurses' home was built in the grounds, so that they no longer had to sleep in rooms adjacent to the wards.

Because infirmaries could be selective over the patients they would admit, it seems that workhouse nurses were of even lower status than those in hospitals, since they were often themselves inmates required to help care for the bedridden paupers or poor women seeking employment. On the other hand, the hundreds of new, purpose-built workhouses in nineteenth-century England meant that their hospital facilities were also new and certainly preferable to the workhouse infirmaries of the Old Poor Law (see Chapter 3). Workhouse nurses, however, were often recorded in considerable detail by visitors, official enquiries and philanthropists concerned at the conditions of the poor. When a new workhouse opened at Gloucester in 1838 the matron's post was advertised in the local press; she was required to be 'A steady, middle-aged woman to undertake the care of the sick in the workhouse, together with lying-in women ... None need apply who are not thoroughly competent to perform the duties'. She was to be paid £30 a year and the nurses £10 10s., with a bonus of £2 2s., a wage-scale also paid at the Gloucester Infirmary. As the first nurse appointed left within a year, the post was advertised, with more specific requirements, in the *Gloucester Journal* on 3 August 1839:

WANTED – a middle-aged active woman as a Nurse to the Gloucester Union. Salary £12 per annum with the usual establishment diet. Testimonials as to character and competence (without which no application will be entertained) to be sent to me at the Workhouse on or before Monday the 12th of August next and personal applications to be made to the Board the following day.
Full particulars as to the nature and extent of the duties required will be given on request to the Master at the Workhouse.

Clerk to the Board.

There were only two applicants for the post, but the woman appointed stayed for nine years. A second nurse was employed by 1848, with an age limit of forty and able to read and write; on this occasion there was only one applicant, who died there in the cholera outbreak of June 1849. When the epidemic raged, the nurse's wage was raised to £15 a year, but it was not until a new hospital was built in 1850 that the nurse was paid £20 annually. By 1879 the Association for Promoting Trained Nurses in Workhouse Infirmaries was formed, but it was not until 1897 that the Central Poor Law Board forbade the employment of paupers as attendants. Not all the medical profession approved of trained nurses in the workhouse and Dr Charles Iliffe at Coventry was representative of this traditional viewpoint. However, more qualified women were being employed in workhouses, and Guardians' minutes increasingly required applicants 'to have undergone for at least three years a course in the medical and surgical wards of a hospital or infirmary'. Nursing was invariably noted by late nineteenth-century Poor Law inspectors as the weakest point in the workhouse, but the ratio of qualified nurses to paupers was to improve the Cinderella service in the last years of the New Poor Law.

It was clear that the status of nursing was to alter as recruits changed from being domestic servants to probationers to pupils, and these changes occurred primarily in the nineteenth-century hospitals. The hospital was essentially a science-based, controlled world, with uniforms of status, and a struggle for control between medical practitioners, administrators and nurses was almost inevitable. The new class of 'lady nurses' were too independent and, especially when encouraged by religious beliefs, could be a formidable force. Their subjugation was, according to The Lancet in 1881, absolutely essential. The emergence of new-style nursing and formal training can be seen from the 1880s and their numbers grew substantially. Before 1861 there were said to be less than a thousand nurses in hospitals; their numbers rose to some 12,500 by the end of the century and in 1905 the figures were 11,038 nurses in voluntary hospitals and some 5000 in poor law institutions. At this period nursing was proving an alternative to other 'white blouse' jobs, such as clerical work and junior school teaching and in 1919 the Nursing Registration Act provided legal definition for the work. The qualification of SRN was to follow.

During these years the basic requirements for becoming a nurse and the duties expected changed considerably, as did the framework in which nurses worked. Women were recruited at a minimum age of twenty-three in voluntary hospitals and at twenty-one in poor law infirmaries, not younger largely because of the physically demanding nature of the work. It was considered that nurses could rarely continue work after the age of thirty-five. Previous experience, especially of housework, was thought valuable. Some hospitals had education tests for nurses, although in the mid-nineteenth century reading a medicine bottle label was the only essential requirement. However, the real problem was the question of who should do menial work in the wards. Hospitals considered that it was character-forming for trainees and that their standards of hygiene would be better for the patients. However, as more middle class women were recruited, the difficulty was only resolved by employing ward orderlies. Nurses' problems were also part of the general political and social climate of the period. Sanitary reform was a major political issue and bad health was seen as a threat to social order, as cholera had recently demonstrated. Hygiene was in addition a further control on working class life and a healthy nation was seen as a powerful one. A further difficulty for nurses was the whole status difference between workhouse hospitals and voluntary infirmaries. With the coming of the New Poor Law patronage shifted from the traditional Overseers to boards of Guardians, who were more likely to be businessmen than landowners, and who would expect the hospitals to be run on the strict principles of less eligibility. The ratio of nurses to patients in the different institutions clearly illustrates this; in voluntary infirmaries it was 1: 3, while in workhouse hospitals it was 1: 20.

As in many other aspects of medicine, the coming of war changed nursing irrevocably. In 1914 it was estimated that 50,000 beds would be needed for service personnel, but in fact by 1918 there were 364,133 beds available, including some requisitioned poor law accommodation. Also in 1914, for a population of thirty-six million, there were only 12,000 trained nurses and about 24,000 medical practitioners. If only as volunteers, in wartime the upper and middle classes gained some knowledge of hospitals and, after three or four months' training, by 1918 there were some 20,000 Voluntary Aid Detachment nurses (VADs) in military hospitals and a further 60,000 in auxiliary hospitals, often experiencing such institutions for the first time.

However, when peace returned, the question for nursing remained – whether nurses should be registered, if nursing should be controlled and by whom? As early as the 1880s there had been moves to found nursing associations, but the establishment of the Ministry of Health in 1919 included nursing as part of its social reforms. Registration meant an identifiable workforce performing a specific service to society but within the profession there was already discord, with the Professional Union of Trained Nurses (founded in 1919) attacking the College of Nursing as an 'employers' combine'. The new Minister of Health, Addison, was concerned at their poor pay, only that of an 'ordinary cook or kitchen maid', but the government would not let nurses be a free professional body, such as law or medicine, and the General Nursing Council became more a certifying than a licensing body, comprising sixteen nurses (only one from a Poor Law institution) and nine lay members.

Overall, demographic and social changes were affecting nurses in the inter-war years; their average age was lower, increased living-in at hospitals discouraged married women and there was a growth in the numbers of orderlies and uncertificated personnel. The Lancet carried out a survey in 1930 showing that nursing was losing popularity as a career to teaching, business and social work for women, at the very time when there was increased demand for their services. Relatively slow to become unionised, although some had joined NALGO, the second world war brought a coherent pattern to nursing. National pay scales appeared in 1941 and terms of service were negotiated under the Rushcliffe Committee, which issued its report on nursing in 1943. Its terms became those for the Whitley Council under the NHS, which saw huge changes in the hospital sector across the country. Nurses, however, remained a minority voice in the new system, with only a handful of their number on the new Regional Hospital Boards and Management Committees. Nurses' pay increased substantially in the early years of the NHS, exceeding the Ministry of Labour's wage index, but status divisions continued, so that in the later 1950s mental hospital nurses were proposing to strike for wages similar to those of their colleagues in other institutions. In 1957 the Nurses' Act abolished the old Supplementary Register and the College allowed men to be recruited. Future requirements on training and negotiations on pay after 1960 have left a profession that Florence Nightingale would not recognise after a hundred and fifty years.

Parish childbirth under the Old Poor Law

	£ s d
1789, parish of Aston Cantlow, Warwickshire	
Mary Hemmings lying in half strike malt	2s. 9d.
Jacob Hemmings wife lying in	2s. 6d.
Man and horse to fetch midwife	2s. 6d.
Wife in labour and want	3s. 0d.
My man and horse to fetch Mr Burman	2s. 6d.
My man and horse with midwife back	2s. 6d.
Midwife for Mary Hemming	5s. 0d.
Turnpike to fetch Mr Burman to Mary Hemming	1d.
Mr Burman for journey and medicines	6s. 0d.
Mary Hemming in want	2s. 0d.
Mary Field for fetching Mr Burman	2s. 6d.
Mr Burman second journey and medicines	£6 15s. 0d.
total	£8 6s. 10d.

Warwickshire County Record Office, DR 259/35

A nursing probationer's day in 1890

7.00 Went on duty. Helped the night nurses' side; washed two patients
7.30 Helped on the day nurses' side; washed a convalescent patient
8.00 Went to prayers
8.15 Washed a typhoid patient
8.15 Washed the urine bottles and the locker tops with chlorinated soda
8.30 Washed and dusted Sister's table and the window ledges. Cleaned and trimmed the lamps. Washed the urine and medicine glasses and small jugs and ...

9.15 Prepared the lunch – bread and milk, served it round

9.45 Went into the bathroom: washed out bath, basins and traps. Put fresh cloths on the ice bowls, folded and put away the clean mattress. Tidied the pillow basket

10.15 Went off duty

11.00 Went to Sister's class

12.45 Went to dinner

1.30 Came on duty. Made beds with Nurse Chaplin. Washed the wine glasses, dusted and tidied the centre of the ward. Put ready the dressing gowns for the doctor

1.50 Cut up 7 lbs of beef for beef tea – made beef tea

2.20 Attended Dr Ord's round and waited on Sister

3.15 Went to Steward's office with a telegraphic message

3.30 Helped Sister to wash an unconscious patient

4.00 Filled three steam kettles

4.20 Cut thin bread and butter for fever patients, prepared tea, served tea round, fed a patient

5.50 Came off duty (tea, 25 minutes)

6.15 Went on duty. Washed specimen glasses, washed feeders, washed gas globes, gave patients their supper

7.15 Made the beds with Nurse Moon

7.45 Tidied the Centre. Arranged and lighted the lamps. Arranged the ink stands.

Took out the flower pots. Turned down the gas

8.00 Carried round the wines and brandies

8.15 Collected the wine glasses

8.30 Came off duty

8.45 Went to prayers

9.00 Had supper

9.20 Went to bed

Privately owned diary

8

INFECTIONS AND DISEASE
CONTROL

[May 1726]
About this time certain remittent and intermittent fevers appeared, particularly
the former, joined in many by pruritus and skin eruptions; which also happened
to other sick people who were not affected in any way by fevers. Almost all the
sick at this time were feverish and complained either of a severe headache or
catarrh of the head and were very prone to delirium and frenzy arising from the
slightest error.

Clifton Wintringham, *Commentarium Nosologicum, a Treatise on
the Study of Diseases*, 3rd edn, 1752

From the earliest times plagues and pestilences had caused widespread suffering
and deaths in Western Europe, some of considerable notoriety, such as the Black
Death in 1349 and the Great Plague of London in 1664–5, in which some 2,000
a week lay dying in August 1665. It was generally accepted that neither formal
nor alternative medicine could help and inhabitants had no natural immunity to
any new infections that came to England. True epidemics attacked all, regardless
of lifestyle, as in the 1918–9 influenza pandemic and even the richest, if afflicted,
could not be saved. Thus Prince Henry, James I's heir, died of typhus in 1612,
while smallpox killed Queen Mary in the epidemic of 1694–5, in which over
2,000 died. Attempts to record causes of death can first be seen in the London
Bills of Mortality from the seventeenth century, although a handful of parish registers occasionally noted why inhabitants had died, presumably because the local
incumbent was interested. Parish registers as such, however, are basically of value
in demographic studies as they provide crude numbers of baptisms, marriages and
burials at a particular church, although epidemics can be suspected in the
increased rate of interments, even though the cause of death is usually not disclosed. Often a better, though non-statistical, view of an epidemic may be gained
from the diaries and correspondence of those living in its midst, who frequently
noted the progress of an infection in the locality and beyond.

However, practitioners cannot have failed to notice sharply rising death rates
in an area, even if they did not attend all those who died. Thus it is surprising

134

how relatively slow physicians and surgeons were to analyse death rates and consider the factors of epidemiology. Apart from Clifton Wintringham, only Joseph Rogers and William Hillary wrote on epidemics in Cork and Ripon respectively at this early period. Clifton Wintringham is thus a remarkably early epidemiologist, who worked all his professional life in York and, for the years 1715–25, noted various epidemics in the area, publishing his findings in 1727. Leaving Cambridge without a medical degree, he settled in Yorkshire where his family had long been yeomen farmers. With a wealthy background and twice marrying well, he clearly had the cream of patients in the area and was able to build a splendid house in the city. He was strongly convinced that climate affected both a disease and the victims' chances of recovery and his *Commentarium* noted outbreaks of measles, smallpox and typhus alongside weather conditions. He thought it was 'sufficiently well known to doctors that certain particular diseases, in a strange way, belong to certain seasons of the year more than to others'. He noted smallpox through the summer and autumn of 1716, putrid fevers at a peak in July and August 1719, with many dead, and indeed Joseph Rogers of Cork was the only other contemporary medical writer to describe the dreadful season of 1718–19. Other epidemics, such as miliary fever in 1727, were exacerbated by the following harsh winter of 1728–9. Although treating an élite clientèle, Wintringham noted that for the 'common people, ... both care of disease and opportunity of medical treatment was lacking'. Fortunately, York parish registers provide excellent support for Wintringham's claims about high mortality rates at certain periods, a topic which later also fascinated Francis Drake, a medical practitioner in the mid century, who analysed death rates across the city.

Smallpox

After bubonic plague had disappeared by the later seventeenth century, smallpox was the most feared, widespread and fatal infection in England, having existed in Western Europe since the late sixth century. In the Tudor and Stuart periods many outbreaks were recorded in England, often beginning in London, as in 1628 and 1634, and spreading to the rest of the country a year later. The disease was passed from one person to another by droplet infection. By the early seventeenth century *variola major* was rife and the London Bills of Mortality show an average of some 2,000 deaths a year. County towns were particularly affected, with outbreaks in Taunton (1658, 1670, 1677, 1684), Cambridge (1674), Bath (1675) and Norwich (1681), for example. Even the greatest in the land were susceptible to the virus; Queen Elizabeth I suffered in the epidemic of 1561–2 and two of Charles I's offspring, the Duke of Gloucester and the Princess of Orange, died from it in 1660.

Although after infection there would have been some degree of maternal and natural immunity in the population at large, smallpox was both endemic and epidemic in the eighteenth century, in spite of the use of inoculation and vaccination. Uniquely it was a disease which permanently scarred the survivor's face ('pockmarked'), as well as a cause of blindness and male infertility. Children were the largest group of deaths and smallpox was undoubtedly a severe check on population growth. In the eighteenth century London experienced eleven peak years, with over 3,000 deaths in each outbreak. There were also country-wide epidemics in the years 1722, 1723 and 1740–2, all clearly reflected in parish burial registers, occasionally annotated by the incumbent. For example, in October 1724, 'The smallpox began about this time and was very fatal throughout the year', while in 1737, another epidemic year, 'The smallpox is ruining my School as fast as it can'. An awareness of the social risk such epidemics posed can be seen in a unique smallpox survey, carried out in the 525 households of Stratford-upon-Avon in April 1765, to enquire who had had smallpox, who had not, whether inoculated and where inhabitants had their legal right of settlement under the Poor Law. Two months later, thirty-one of the town's thirty-six burials were smallpox victims. A similar but less detailed survey was carried out at Brighton in 1786, resulting in the inoculation of 1,887 unprotected inhabitants.

As the largest community in Britain, London's smallpox problems were considerable. The city had some exceptionally poor areas, as well as the grandest houses and the most medical practitioners in the kingdom. John Coakley Lettsom, the Quaker physician, could comment that 'most born in London have smallpox before they are seven' and certainly the eighteenth-century statistical evidence for the capital is extensive; Lettsom considered it reliable, as a disease 'which the most ignorant cannot easily mistake for another'. The year 1723 marked the capital's smallpox peak for the first half-century, with 3,271 deaths (11 per cent), although a mild version of the disease, but surpassed in the years 1750–1800 by 1772 (3,992 deaths, or 15 per cent) and 1796 (3,548 deaths, or 18 per cent). In fact, the last two decades of the century showed a lower death rate from all causes in London, suggesting that the general state of health was improving for whatever reasons.

Smallpox can increasingly be seen in the old large cities and new industrial centres, where it persisted, but leaving market towns and villages, with longer intervals between outbreaks. Thus there were 2,700 deaths in Edinburgh (nearly 7 per cent) in the two years 1740–42, primarily children under five, while in Leeds in 1781, with a population of some 17,000, smallpox was the cause of 130 deaths out of 462 (28 per cent). Manchester suffered six years of continuous smallpox, 1769–74, with a peak in 1771, virtually all children under the age of five, and a death rate of 15.3 per cent from the disease; a further disastrous outbreak occurred, as at Leeds, in 1781. In contrast, at Boston, a medium-sized market town, in the years 1769–1800, although there were four epidemics (1770, 1775, 1784, 1796), there were thirteen years with no smallpox deaths recorded and eleven years when deaths from the infection were in single figures. Creighton cites various other small towns in England with similar statistics and local newspapers regularly carried reports declaring that a particular community was free of smallpox. The sudden arrival of those with smallpox would frequently cause an epidemic, as at Plymouth in 1751, when the disease was brought into the town by 'Conway's regiment' and was then prevalent there for two years. Foreign travel was also a threat to those with no immunity, including young gentlemen on the Grand Tour; thus the Marquess of Rockingham noted in 1734 'my eldest son Thomas died of smallpox at Leyden'.

Smallpox, however, is the first disease, and for over a century the only one, where medical intervention, rather than government action, actually caused a decline in deaths. Clearly, a higher standard of living was always helpful in patients' resistance and recovery but inoculation and vaccination were medical techniques to prevent an infection, rather than treatment when illness had occurred or relying on a raised natural immunity. Even before the activities of Lady Mary Wortley Montagu, accounts of 'ingrafting' or 'transplantation' to prevent smallpox in the Middle East had been circulating among the British medical profession. Inoculation in fact involved deliberately infecting a healthy person with smallpox 'matter' (pus) put into a cut from another individual who was suffering only a mild form of the disease. Thus the newly-inoculated patient would survive a lesser attack and be immune in future. John Woodward MD of London described the technique at a meeting of the Royal Society and his account was published in the *Philosophical Transactions* of 1714. A similar custom was also apparently known in Welsh folk-medicine from the early seventeenth century. When Lady Wortley Montagu returned to England in 1718 from Constantinople, where her husband was British ambassador, her infant son had already been inoculated there and in 1721, a smallpox epidemic year in London, her young daughter was also inoculated. The Princess of Wales, anxious to have her own children protected, persuaded George I to have the technique tried out on six felons at Newgate prison, whose capital sentences were remitted as a reward; all survived. After eleven charity children were also successfully treated, the two young princesses were inoculated under the direction of Sir Hans Sloane, the royal physician. In 1723 a total of 292 people were inoculated and the technique became increasingly popular, until deaths began to be reported. It cannot have encouraged inoculations for Londoners to read in the press in 1725:

> March 16, died Mrs Eyles, niece of Sir John Eyles, alderman of London, of the smallpox contracted by inoculation. June 17, died of the small-pox contracted by inoculation, Arthur Hill, esquire, eldest son of Viscount Hilsborough. August 12, died of the smallpox by inoculation, — Hurst, of Salisbury, esquire.

In fact, Creighton is convinced that virtually no inoculations took place in England in the period from 1728 to 1740, until a milder form of the virus had been used in Charleston, South Carolina, and the practitioner responsible there, James Kirkpatrick MD, came to London and published his findings. Certainly by the 1740s many medical practitioners of repute, such as Mead, Sloane and Arbuthnot, pronounced in favour of the technique. However, there were always professionally divergent views and William Bromfield, the royal surgeon, gave up inoculating altogether, while John Barker of Coleshill could write of smallpox in 1769 as no more than a 'bugbear'.

However, until the middle years of the eighteenth century, inoculation remained an expensive procedure, restricted to the wealthy. It was also a lucrative part of medical practice, performed by some of the leading London consultants. Gentry family accounts frequently contain expenses for inoculating members of the family and servants, both in the country and in London. The difference in professional fees, depending on the status of the patient, was marked. Thus, in 1786 Walter Farquhar, a famous London practitioner, was paid £10 10s. for inoculating a gentleman's young daughter when they were visiting the capital and four years later the same gentleman spent £7 15s. for inoculating thirty-one poor (5s. each) near his Herefordshire estate. Before inoculation took place the prosperous patient was required to be purged, bled and on a 'low' diet (no animal foods or alcohol), and this automatically made the process costly. One patient, treated by Robert Sutton at Newark in 1767, spent three weeks on the procedure and was charged five guineas, noting 'inoculation has been practised in this country and so much and with so great success, that it seems to have lost all its terrors'. However, it was apparent that when the poor caught smallpox they not only infected the prosperous but caused parish spending to rise disastrously. Some parishes maintained an isolation building for victims. Overseers of the Poor responded by paying for inoculations for their parishioners, both individually and en masse, using medical practitioners and lay inoculators. Thus in 1772 at Shipston-on-Stour, a market town with some two hundred families, a local surgeon contracted to inoculate 157 poor inhabitants at 6s. a head, a cost to the ratepayers of £37 12s. 6d. Later in the century inoculation was carried out on an even larger scale, 738 at Painswick in 1786, 1,215 at Luton in the same year and some 500 at Bocking for only £5 in 1790, for example, and both Baron Dimsdale and Daniel Sutton undertook parish work. Free inoculation was also provided through charities, the earliest of which was the London Smallpox and Inoculation Hospital, founded in 1746. In the provinces dispensaries were established for this purpose at Whitehaven, Bath, Newcastle upon Tyne, Chester, Carlisle and Liverpool, where over five hundred inoculations were carried out in its first year, 1781.

Among the inoculators, the Sutton family were undoubtedly the most influential, running a partnership franchise system, selling the secrets of their particular technique to other medical practitioners round the country for either an initial fee (£50 to £100) or a half share of profits. By 1754 the College of Physicians could pronounce inoculation as 'highly salutary to the human race' and the Suttons' efforts were considerable in its wide acceptance. Robert Sutton, a Suffolk surgeon, began inoculating in about 1757 and was advertising his services by 1762, using a method 'done without Incision'. In ten years, 1757–67, he had inoculated 2,514 patients, using the month-long preparation technique. His son, Daniel, broke from his father in 1763 and set up in practice on his own in

Ingatestone, where he boarded patients. In his first year he made £2,100 and in 1765 this sum trebled; during the period 1764–6 he inoculated 13,792 patients, while his assistants treated a further six hundred. He claimed that there were no deaths from his method. In fact, the Suttonian technique, as had been used in Turkey, relied on using smallpox matter from a recent and mild attack, which never produced a severe reaction. Daniel Sutton also considerably reduced the preparation and residence time for patients, claiming that there seemed no adverse reactions if there were no preparation at all. In 1796 he wrote that 'it has been a practice of late, to give up preparation, medicinal and dietetic entirely'. The Suttons were, in fact, very businesslike in their activities. There were six sons and two sons-in-law of Robert Sutton who practised as inoculators and by 1768 there were forty-five 'Suttonians' in twenty-six English counties, as well as two in Wales, nine in Ireland, two in Paris, two in The Hague and two in the West Indies, providing considerable coverage. These partnerships were invariably advertised in the local press, often including the numbers of patients inoculated; thus Mr Milbourne claimed to have attended over 20,000 in the Coventry area by 1771. However, by the late 1770s there were numbers of lay and medical practitioners offering a cheaper service than the Suttons'; and by the last years of the century inoculation was actively practised only in the countryside and in those large towns where there were charitable provisions.

The Suttons' main rival was Thomas Dimsdale, created Baron Dimsdale by Catherine the Great after he had visited Russia in 1768 to inoculate the Empress, her children, servants and members of the imperial court. As well as a fee of £10,000 and £2,000 expenses, he also received an annuity of £500 and the title by which he was usually known. In his *Present Method of Inoculating for the Smallpox* (1767), a widely popular book, he advocated reducing the preparation time for inoculating and wrote of his own experiences in mass inoculations in the villages near his home town of Hertford, a theme he developed later in *Thoughts on General and Partial Inoculation* (1776). Dimsdale claimed to have lost only one patient from an inoculation in over two decades and insisted that even a higher death-rate from the technique was only 'a cypher' in contrast to the deaths that occurred from natural smallpox. The importance attached to inoculation by the public is reflected in contemporary letters and diaries, where the event is frequently recorded. It is clear that writers saw inoculation of their children as a parental duty, often recording their fears at the risks attached. Some, like Abigail Gawthern of Nottingham, simply noted the date of her young daughter's inoculation in 1784, while the Revd Woodforde gave a detailed account when his two servants were treated in 1776, with prayers for their recovery.

The name of Edward Jenner is amongst the most famous in British history for his discovery of vaccination, yet it was not until he had practised for twenty-five years that his work was widely known. Jenner was apprenticed to a local surgeon-apothecary, George Hardwick of Chipping Sodbury, for seven years in 1765 at the age of sixteen with the substantial premium of £100. He then spent some time at St George's Hospital, London as a pupil of John Hunter, with whom he remained in contact after returning to Gloucestershire to begin practice at Berkeley in 1772. He developed an interest in discovering why inoculation was not always effective and collected over a thousand instances of such failures. In his daily practice in a dairying county, he had noticed that milkmaids and stockmen handling cows rarely developed smallpox, even if not inoculated, when an epidemic struck and he presumed that cowpox, which these workers had caught, was in some way a substitute for smallpox. Benjamin Jesty, a Yetminster farmer, had already noticed this link in 1774, but did not follow it through. Jenner experimented by inoculating a village lad, eight-year-old James Phipps, with cowpox and then, six weeks later, with smallpox, which did not develop. Jenner wrote a short paper on the discovery in 1798, *An Enquiry into the Causes and Effects of the Variola Vaccinae*, as well as vaccinating more inhabitants with cowpox. There were immediate objections to his proposals; the inoculators predictably attacked his technique for fear of losing their livelihoods, the clergy preached against the use of an animal infection in humans and vaccination became the butt for cartoonists, including Gillray. Whereas inoculation could protect the individual but also spread smallpox, there were no such risks with vaccination, because the bovine virus was not malignant.

Among the medical supporters of Jenner's method was John Coakley Lettsom, who had always approved of mass inoculation, and in 1802 a Committee of the House of Commons met to consider Jenner's work. Jenner was rewarded with the gift of £10,000 from the King and a further £20,000 five years later. Vaccination was soon preferred to inoculation, so that some 100,000 people had been vaccinated by 1801; in 1807 parliament required the Royal College of Physicians to organise vaccination supplies across the country and the National Vaccine Establishment was set up a year later. Vaccinations were advertised in the local press from an early period, using 'genuine cowpox matter', and parish authorities spent considerable sums on mass vaccinations. However, inoculation was often preferred in remote rural areas, in spite of the risk of infection from one person to another and although a prison sentence could be imposed for its use. In 1814 there had been discussions about compulsory vaccination of the poor, but the smallpox epidemic of 1837–40, with 35,000 deaths, especially of poor children, decided the matter. *The Lancet* blamed inoculation for the high death rate and the government declared it a felony in 1840, requiring children to be vaccinated at the ratepayers' expense, if their parents agreed. An Act of 1867 authorised Boards of Guardians to enforce infant vaccination. A severe smallpox epidemic in 1870–1 resulted in the appointment of Public Vaccinators and the last major outbreak occurred in 1902–3. A conscience clause allowed parents who resisted vaccination for their children to appeal to two JPs and compulsion ended in 1948. No epidemic has been reported in England since 1934, although single cases have been imported as a result of foreign travel or from laboratory accidents.

Many other advances in vaccinations have been made as a result of Jenner's discovery that viral and other infections could be halted by immunisation, beginning with Pasteur's vaccine against rabies. Above all, however, apart from better public sewerage, smallpox is a striking example of a disease eradicated firstly by private medical intervention and later by government action and has been called 'a landmark in social history'.

Tuberculosis

Tuberculosis can rightly be claimed as the disease of antiquity, for evidence of infection has been found in Egyptian tombs and its medical name, phthisis, is from a Greek word meaning 'wasting', hence the general term 'consumption'. Recognised as an affliction of young adults and well described by Galen, man was susceptible to only two of the five kinds of tuberculosis, human and bovine. A bacterial infection and strongly familial, the external factors that promoted its spread – a low standard of living and even occupational risks – were not recognised until the later nineteenth century. In *De Phthysi* (1685), John Locke wrote that a fifth of all deaths in London were from consumption, a disease from which he suffered and which killed his father and brother. The London Bills of Mortality support this estimate. His work was followed four years later by Richard Morton's important survey of pulmonary tuberculosis, noting the symptoms of inappetence, amenorrheoea and extreme wasting.

One of the commonest forms of the disease was scrofula, tubercular glands of the neck, known as the King's Evil which certain European monarchies were believed to have sacred powers of healing. Shakespeare noted the phenomenon in *Macbeth* (Act IV, scene 3) and Charles II is said to have 'touched' 92,102 sufferers in his twenty-five-year reign, although the ceremony ceased after the death of the last Stuart monarch, Queen Anne. However, pulmonary tuberculosis was by far a greater cause of deaths and many early medical writers noted its various aspects; Paracelsus commented on miners' phthisis after he had visited Cornwall, Fracastorius stressed its genetic factor in *De Contagione* (1546) and it was clearly of interest to both Thomas Willis and Thomas Sydenham in the seventeenth century.

Tuberculosis was, unfortunately, frequently misdiagnosed and even confused with other infections, but Boerhaave's invention of the thermometer enabled its fever to be identified; later, percussion of the chest with the stethoscope was devised by Laënnac, (who himself died of the disease) to make accurate diagnosis of pulmonary tuberculosis possible. Apart from quack remedies, standard treatments included a low diet and regular blood-letting, a technique which was to last until the mid-nineteenth century, although Laënnec's view that 'it never cured a single case of consumption' found little professional support. Laudanum (morphine) was the single effective means of suppressing the cough and removing the pain of the latter stages of the disease and was widely used.

The disease had long been associated with artists and writers, such as Watteau and Laurence Sterne in the eighteenth century, with Keats and the Brontës perhaps the best-known examples in the nineteenth. However, a recent writer has noted that tuberculosis was 'generally deeply respectful of wealth and rank', emphasising that overcrowding and poor diet were important contributory factors. Increasingly, a moral argument came to be made that associated tuberculosis with depravity and indulgence, as well as with spiritual anguish and depression. The disease reached a peak and became endemic in England in the years 1780–1830 and, when a Registrar General was appointed and accurate statistics became available in 1839, tuberculosis was shown to be responsible for 17.6 per cent of all deaths. The highest death rates were in London and the great industrial towns, with an average of 60,000 deaths a year in the period 1839–43, falling to 51,000 in 1851–5. By the end of the century tuberculosis deaths had dropped to 10.4 per cent of the total, but it was still prominent in the table of causes of death, second only to heart disease. At this period it was the most fatal of all diseases in England; there was an overall decline in mortality in the period 1840–1900 and the incidence of tuberculosis continued to fall until 1914.

At this period effective treatment simply did not exist, although digitalis and tartar emetic were widely used, and even the famous Erasmus Darwin struggled with a bizarre range of remedies when he was treating the young daughter of James Watt for some six months before her death in 1794. There was predictably a wide range of quack cures, including a country belief in inhaling the warm breath of farm animals, a myth that may have been linked to the bovine form of tuberculosis. General hospitals all excluded consumptive patients. In medical circles there was a growing interest in inhalation for pulmonary tuberculosis, led by the experiments of Thomas Beddoes MD at Bristol, where he founded his Pneumonic Medical Institution in the 1790s, using pure gases for the purpose. To attempt to treat scrofula, Lettsom set up his Royal Sea Bathing Infirmary at Margate in 1791, relying on the fresh coastal breezes. A virtually unknown Warwickshire practitioner, George Bodington, devised a regime for sufferers that, many years later, would be widely adopted, namely fresh cool air and light exercise. In the 1840s he established what would later be considered a sanatorium in Sutton Coldfield, where he also ran a private lunatic asylum. In 1840 he published *An Essay on the Treatment and Cure of Pulmonary Consumption*, advocating 'the free use of a pure atmosphere', with mild exercise, walking or riding, and good food, preferably living in a separate house in a 'high and dry' rural location. His publication was immediately derided by the medical profession and his views were not supported until 1890, when the American Dr E. L. Trudeau took up Bodington's findings and became famous in the process. However, Bodington's obituary notice in *The Lancet* in 1882 rather belatedly acknowledged the work of this 'simple village doctor' as 'among the first to advocate the more rational, scientific and successful treatment of pulmonary consumption which we now practise'.

In the year of Bodington's death, in Germany Robert Koch isolated the tubercle bacillus and identified it as the specific organism of pulmonary tuberculosis, later followed by the use of tuberculin as a skin test to determine whether a patient had ever had the disease and was still at risk. The use of X-rays, discovered in 1895 by Karl Willhelm Röntgen, had made diagnosis easier, although a hazardous procedure for many years to come. The national pattern of tuberculosis changed by the early twentieth century and in 1901 the highest death rates (over 1,400 per million) could be seen in Northumberland, Yorkshire, Warwickshire and Wales, but much lower (1,000 per million) in the Welsh borders, Hampshire and Oxfordshire. It became a notifiable disease in 1913, a year in which there were 117,000 cases and 5,000 deaths in England and Wales. Numbers of sanatoria grew, initially privately-run, but the Manchester Sanatorium at Bowden set the pattern for many later ones to follow. There were eighty-four in Britain by 1911, providing about 8,000 beds, although some Poor Law authorities, such as Bradford and Liverpool, had already built their own sanatoria, while some general hospitals, as at Sheffield, provided special open-air accommodation for tuberculosis cases. As a result of government intervention £1.5m was provided in 1911 through Lloyd George's National Insurance Act for the construction of sanatoria and by 1930 there were 500 establishments providing 25,000 beds.

The establishment of villages or colonies for tuberculosis patients was a new development in the inter-war years Some, however, were earlier, such as the institution at Munsley in Norfolk, built in 1899, with Swiss-style hillside chalets for working and middle class patients. Perhaps the most famous development was that at Papworth, near Cambridge, founded in 1916, which, as well as treating sufferers from the disease, was also an industrial village that provided instruction in crafts and trades so that patients were rehabilitated and could earn their livelihoods. They spent eighteen hours a day in the open air. In 1921 the Public Health (Tuberculosis) Act (11 and 12 Geo. V, c. 12) provided treatment for all, even if they were not insured under Lloyd George's scheme. However, until the 1940s tuberculosis was the commonest cause of death in young adults. With the coming of streptomycin in 1953 as an effective antibiotic therapy, new surgical techniques, BCG vaccinations and the widespread use of chest X-rays for early diagnosis, especially mobile units, tuberculosis had been in steady decline for four decades by the 1980s. In the years 1982–93, however, some 6,000 cases were recorded, with new drug-resistant strains closely linked to complacency in medication by patients. In 1998 some 6,000 cases were reported in Britain.

Typhus

As England was becoming free from plague, although there were still occasional outbreaks in Queen Elizabeth's reign, typhus, 'the new disease' became a major cause of deaths across Stuart England, particularly in towns. It was transmitted by lice and fleas and was essentially a winter disease that thrived in dirty, poor living conditions. However, with low natural immunity, in the early seventeenth century even the wealthy were its victims; James I's heir, Prince Henry, died from typhus in London in November 1612, attended by Sir Theodore Mayerne, who later wrote a treatise, *Ad Febrem Purpuream*, on the disease. Death was often very sudden; the Duke of Lennox died within three days of becoming ill and many sufferers succumbed to heart failure before the distinctive typhus rash appeared. A particularly serious outbreak in 1623–4 caused parliament to adjourn and some later epidemics affected the progress of the Civil War, as at Reading in 1643 and at Tiverton a year later.

Typhus, however, is best known for its high death rate in the eighteenth century, when it was referred to as 'gaol fever' or 'factory fever'. There had in fact been earlier outbreaks in prisons, usually nicknamed as Black Assizes, as at Cambridge in 1522, Oxford in 1577 and Exeter in 1586, when attorneys died alongside felons and in 1750, when infection occurred at the Old Bailey, there were some fifty deaths, including a judge and the Lord Mayor of London. Ventilators were designed for prisons, but changes in 1746 to the Window Tax meant that fresh air was reduced wherever possible to save money. Across the country, a number of outbreaks followed years of particularly bad harvests (1718, 1722, 1741–2) and by later in the century the large industrial towns, such as Newcastle, Leeds, Liverpool and Hull, recorded high death rates from typhus, while in Manchester in 1773 mortality was twice that in the nearby villages. The local press usually noted such epidemics and at Leeds in January 1779, for example, the *Mercury* reported that 'putrid fever was prevailing in the Leeds area'.

Medical treatment was invariably ineffectual and this can be seen in practitioners' own case notes, such as those kept by William Brownrigg MD of Whitehaven, who was convinced that certain fevers were related to specific times of the year. The fatality rate of typhus is best illustrated in the deaths of practitioners who themselves succumbed to the disease. In the Lancashire outbreak of 1750–1, four of the immediate family of Richard Kay, a surgeon-apothecary, died in the epidemic of 'spotted fever', which also caused Kay's death at the age of thirty-five. When John Howard travelled the country visiting various prisons, he noted that typhus had caused the deaths of gaol surgeons at Bedford, Warwick and Worcester. In its other manifestation, typhus was also known as 'factory fever' and became a topic of great public anxiety when an outbreak occurred in Peel's cotton factory at Radcliffe, near Manchester, in 1784 and began to spread into the locality.

Typhus, under its great variety of names, including workhouse, pestilential, nervous and putrid fever, continued to be both epidemic and endemic in the early nineteenth century, an 'unerring index of destitution', with severe outbreaks in 1817–19, 1826–7, 1831–2, 1837 and 1846–8, the first of which struck at virtually every town and village in England. The market town of Banbury provides an interesting example of the death rates during the years 1817–22 (100, 132, 139, 128, 126, 111). In this period, infants and children suffered most, so that in the peak year, 1819, they formed 41 per cent of all deaths, some only a day old, although surprisingly there were also burials of eight octogenarians from the town. The 1837 epidemic, which caused the deaths of 6,011 in London in eighteen months, also afflicted country towns, and in this year there were 154 burials in Banbury, which fell to the normal level of 111 in the following year. As well as the great towns of the North, other areas also had serious outbreaks, including Wolverhampton, Dudley, Swansea, Macclesfield and Norwich. The next epidemic of 1846–7 was thought to have come from Irish immigrants who fled their potato crop failure and was known as 'famine fever'. Fever cases, of course, had always been excluded from general hospitals and it was not until charitable Houses of Recovery were built, as at Liverpool in 1801, or special fever wards, as at Manchester in 1796, that typhus cases could be nursed outside the home. However, there was a sharp fall in the death rate from typhus, originally responsible for about a fifth of all deaths, from the middle of the nineteenth century onwards, with sanitary improvements a critical factor in its reduction.

Cholera

Although cholera was known to English travellers in the eighteenth century, it did not spread into Europe from Asia until the middle years of the nineteenth. The causative organism was *vibrio cholerae*, identified by Koch in 1883, and human beings were its host, but water-borne bacteria were the commonest cause of infection. It particularly thrived in high temperatures, low-lying land, ponds and lakes and in these conditions it had been endemic in the Indian sub-continent from ancient times. Prevalent in such great cities as Moscow and Paris and moving across Europe at about five miles a day, it was spread by faeces in person to person contact and in water contaminated by a sufferer's faeces. It was extremely contagious, rapid in its onset and with a very high fatality rate; death from dehydration usually occurred within two to six days. Britain was not affected until the second great nineteenth-century cholera pandemic of 1831. In that year it was first seen in Sunderland on 19 October and spread along the banks of the Tyne. Thence through Northumberland, the epidemic turned north into Scotland, with 3,166 deaths in Glasgow, and south to Yorkshire and Lancashire. In these counties too fatalities were high, with 702 deaths in Leeds, 185 in York, 1,523 in Liverpool and 706 in Manchester. Cholera arrived in February 1832 in London, where there were 5,275 deaths. The industrial Midlands suffered particularly, with 1,870 deaths in Staffordshire, 693 of which were in Bilston and 281 in Tipton. However, although few counties escaped an outbreak, some rural areas had only a few deaths, for example, Derbyshire (16), Wiltshire (14), Leicestershire (5) and Suffolk (1), while in Herefordshire, Sussex, Northamptonshire and Rutland none was reported. Total deaths totalled 21,882 in England and Wales out of a population of nearly 14 million. As a disease cholera was fairly class-specific, with many fatalities among a town's poorest inhabitants and notably in institutions, asylums, workhouses and prisons; unlike typhus, medical immunity to cholera was remarkable. When an outbreak occurred a few miles from Eton College in July 1832, with five deaths, pupils' parents were urged to take their sons home before the vacation was due to begin. They were assured, however, that 'every precaution has been taken of covering the bodies with lime and committing them to an extra deep grave the same day, lime-washing the houses and fumigating or dressing the clothes, etc.'.

Government action to control epidemics had been planned nearly thirty years earlier in 1804, when it seemed that yellow fever might enter Britain and the first national Board of Health was established. As there was then no outbreak of yellow fever after all, the Board was dissolved in 1806, never having functioned. However, on 21 June 1831 a Central Board of Health was created, largely composed of medical consultants and senior military men, to prepare rules that would guard against cholera, the first time that public health was to be controlled by local and central government. In every town and village boards of health were set up, consisting of leading local figures, including medical practitioners; premises were to be provided where cholera victims could be taken and sufferers' possessions were to be cleansed or burnt. Special burial grounds were designated in many towns, where the old graveyards were too full for so many new interments. Victims were to be visited by a local practitioner and the committee members' names were publicly displayed. The army and police were to enforce the rules when necessary. The editor of *The Lancet* raged against the restrictions.

However, when cholera reached Hamburg on 12 October, these rules were acknowledged as necessary and the Home Secretary instructed JPs to see that they were followed. Local Boards were established in over twenty-five towns by mid-November and experienced medical practitioners were added to the Central Board. By the end of the epidemic in December 1832 there were some 820 local Boards of Health in England and Wales. However, political factors became intertwined with medical considerations, as 1832 saw agitation for parliamentary reform and for drastic changes to the Old Poor Law. In July 1842 Edwin Chadwick published his *Report of an Inquiry into the Sanitary Conditions of the Labouring Population of Great Britain*; the word 'sanitary' was newly-coined for the report. In 1844 the *Report of the Health of Towns* appeared, followed by the first Public Health Act four years later. In public health reforms Liverpool led the way, in 1847 appointing the first Medical Officer of Health in Britain, as well as a Borough Engineer and Inspector of Nuisances; other authorities later followed this example, installing sewerage systems and good water supplies, often in the face of local opposition at such expenditure.

Not surprisingly, the cholera epidemic created fear and even panic in the population at large, clearly illustrated in contemporary cartoons (Figure 8.1), and in December 1831 one Norwich general practitioner wrote to a colleague of:

> The cholerophobia prevailing to an extreme degree and Boards of Health established with a determination to starve out the disease should it invade us ... so if the cholera do not spread, the fear of it will bring general good by leading to such sanitary measures as ought always to be in force.

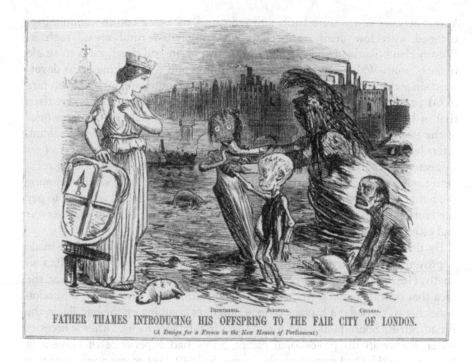

FATHER THAMES INTRODUCING HIS OFFSPRING TO THE FAIR CITY OF LONDON.
(A Design for a Fresco in the New Houses of Parliament.)

Figure 8.1 A *Punch* cartoon on the pollution of the River Thames, 1858

In fact, 129 died of cholera in Norwich out of a total of 232 deaths in the county. In the same outbreak, Thomas Smart, a Berkshire surgeon-apothecary, noted cholera as 'threatening to devastate our country' and described how he himself treated the disease with 'brandy and opium, stimulating frictions to the body, stimulating injections, and the hot sand-bath'. He also recommended injections of carbolic acid or natural salts, as well as transfusions of healthy blood. The salts therapy is very similar to the saline technique now used in treating the disease and the topic received some discussion in the contemporary *London Medical Gazette*. Services of thanksgiving were held across the country when the epidemic had waned.

The next cholera epidemic did not reach England from India until the autumn of 1848, beginning simultaneously at Newhaven and Edinburgh and spreading to the rest of the country by June 1849. In a more severe outbreak than that of 1831–2, with a total of 53,293 deaths in England and Wales, there were again striking differences between death rates in various counties. Apart from London, with 14,137 deaths (6.2 per 1,000), the East Riding of Yorkshire, particularly Hull, was worst affected, with 2,140 deaths (8.7 per 1,000), although the Black Country again experienced a severe outbreak (1,365 died in the Wolverhampton area), as did ports such as Plymouth (830) and Bristol (591). Whereas the

Yorkshire wool towns were badly affected, the Lancashire cotton communities escaped with low death rates. The less populated rural areas, such as Westmorland, Rutland and Herefordshire, also again had death rates in single figures. South Wales, especially the new mining and ironworking areas developed since the 1832 epidemic, had a particularly bad outbreak, with a death rate of 6.1 per thousand. It is clear that the 1849 epidemic was far more severe than that of 1832, but again struck the large towns, even if not always the same ones as the first epidemic. Demands for better water supplies arose all over England, often led by the clergy. Thus the Revd Patrick Brontë secured the visit of an inspector, B. H. Babbage, to Haworth in 1850 as a result of petitioning for a better water supply, pleading that 'there has been a great deal of sickness among us', but he lacked the support of the leading inhabitants, who did not wish to pay the costs of piped water. His parishioners had to wait eight years for a reservoir and clean water supply.

By the time the 1853–4 epidemic arrived in Britain, most areas had made improvements; the highest death rate was again in London, with over half of all deaths (10,738 out of a total of 20,097). Most medical opinion still resisted the idea that contaminated water caused cholera, until John Snow MD, a London anaesthetist, carried out his famous experiment of chaining up the handle on the Broad Street, Soho, pump and forcing the inhabitants to use other sources of water. Earlier in his professional career Snow had experience of cholera at Newcastle and he had written on the disease in 1849. He became convinced that water tainted with sewage was the cause of the 344 deaths in four days among those using the Broad Street well. Snow's work provided proof that cholera was a water-borne infection that could be controlled by a pure water supply and good sewerage. Substantial sums had been spent on sewerage systems in the 1850s, £8,519 in York, for example, although half of this amount had provided facilities to one of the city's wealthiest areas.

Inspectors of Nuisances were also a force in improving town living conditions. A major step forward in public health was undoubtedly the appointment of local Medical Officers of Health. The first was William Henry Duncan in Liverpool in 1847, whose pioneering efforts reduced the town's high infant mortality and improved housing generally. A powerful element in reform was the work of John Simon, London's first Medical Officer of Health, and the Registrar General's recently-appointed statistician, William Farr. They studied the figures for the 1849 and 1853 outbreaks, comparing the supplies of two water companies, Lambeth and Southwark. Their findings showed a striking difference between the two, with Southwark's water condemned as 'perhaps the filthiest stuff ever drunk by a civilised community'. In 1848 The Times could comment that 'The Cholera is the best of all sanitary reformers, it overlooks no mistake and pardons no oversight'.

The fourth and final cholera epidemic was brought to England in 1865–6 by emigrants from Europe en route to America, travelling from the east coast ports to Liverpool, where the outbreak was severe, with 2,122 deaths. No county except Rutland escaped infection and, although there were 14,378 deaths in all, fatalities were low and were widely dispersed across the country, largely due to greatly improved public health systems. Only in the East End of London were death rates comparable to those of 1849, while all the other great centres of infection remained lightly affected.

Typhoid

The causative organism of typhoid, *salmonella typhi*, transmitted by water, milk and contaminated food, was endemic in England throughout the eighteenth and early nineteenth centuries and its enteric fever was a common cause of death. Although it was declining with improved water supplies, better sewerage and greater personal hygiene, there was a significantly lower death rate only after 1871. Although typhoid was closely linked to poor living conditions, even the highest in the land could become infected, so that Prince Albert is thought to have died from it in 1861 and the Prince of Wales was seriously ill a decade later, although positive diagnosis of typhoid was not always possible. Typhoid formed a crucial part of the plot in several novels of Charlotte M. Yonge, especially *The Daisy Chain*, *The Young Stepmother* and *The Three Brides*, with one of her characters stating that 'defective drains were as dangerous to the upper classes as the absence of drains to the lower'. Typhoid was exacerbated by the presence in many larger communities of inner-city slaughter houses, the Shambles of the medieval period, and these too had to be re-sited outside city limits, as at York.

However, it is undeniable that clean water and better sanitation increased life expectancy, which in 1841 had been forty for a boy and forty-two for a girl, although social class and geography made a great deal of difference. Greater longevity was the result, with a million inhabitants over sixty-five in 1852, but five million by 1951, when over a third of all households in Britain still lacked a fixed bath and some 8 per cent had no flushing lavatory.

Influenza

The influenza virus, commonest in winter, spread by droplet infection via the respiratory tract, has been called 'the last plague' of the modern world, 'an unchanging disease due to a changing virus'. In spite of its altered virulence across the centuries, its essential characteristics of short duration, suddenly arriving and departing, remained the same, but generally thriving in winter due to closer living conditions. There had been influenza epidemics identified in England in the Tudor period, but the pandemic of 1580 was comparable to only the disastrous worldwide outbreak of 1918–19. In the second half of the seventeenth century, when there was an epidemic each decade, it was known as the new fever or new ague.

The first half of the eighteenth century witnessed five outbreaks of influenza, as did the years 1750–1800 (1762, 1767, 1775, 1782 and 1788). In April 1762, it was noted that the infection in London 'pervaded the whole city, far and wide, scarcely sparing anyone' and the long-lasting symptoms, familiar to modern sufferers, were sweating, languor of body and depression of spirits. More is known of the 1775 epidemic because John Fothergill distributed questionnaires to practitioners requesting details of influenza in their particular areas. This outbreak had low death rates, although nowhere escaped; thus all but two of the 175 patients in Exeter hospital were infected, as were all 175 inhabitants of the House of Industry at Chester, where John Howard found prisoners in the gaol ill with the disease. However, it was in the relatively mild pandemic of 1782 that the College of Physicians first called this particular disease influenza, although the word had earlier been used of outbreaks in Italy before they reached England. The 1782 epidemic, spreading from Asia, through Russia and into Northern Europe, reached Newcastle upon Tyne, thence to London and the eastern counties by June. Some 75 to 80 per cent of the population were affected, although children and the elderly were spared. Although influenza was not named as the cause of illness, raised spending by the Overseers of the Poor, often by as much as a third, is striking in their annual accounts, even in remote rural parishes.

Although influenza epidemics occurred again in England in 1803, 1831, 1833 and 1847–8, they received little medical or other comment, although the last of these outbreaks could be accurately assessed for the first time in history since registration of deaths had begun in 1839. Medical opinion still considered it noncontagious. However, the outbreaks of 1889–94 were the first of the modern influenza pandemics, precursors to that of 1918–19 in many respects. Influenza reached Britain by January 1890, at that time still in a fairly mild form, having been reported in the early winter of 1889 in most European capitals, its more rapid spread greatly helped by the new railway networks across the continent. Known as Russian flu, and caused by mutation of the A-type virus, it returned three more times, with the second wave, early in 1891, as the most serious, with high death rates, in Sheffield, Bradford and Huddersfield, for example, although the south-east was badly affected in 1892 and the Midlands in 1893. This epidemic was unique in that the original outbreak revived in more lethal form in three successive seasons.

The epidemic that ranks closest to the Black Death, however, occurred at the end of the first World War, when influenza caused more deaths than trench warfare. The first wave of a new strain, known as Spanish flu, arrived in Britain in May to July of 1918, followed by a more severe outbreak in October and November. A third wave appeared in February 1919, again particularly killing those in the twenty to forty age group with no immunity, rather than the elderly; the civilian population was exhausted by four years of war and poor nutrition, while demobilised servicemen returning home were particularly affected. Some 200,000 died in England and Wales and the whole post-war economic recovery was certainly adversely affected by the outbreak. The most recent great pandemics of influenza in England were in 1957–8, known as Asian flu, and in 1968 when Hong Kong flu reached this country, but in both outbreaks mortality was far lower than in 1918–19.

Venereal diseases

Of the two commonest sexually transmitted diseases, gonorrhoea and syphilis, only the latter was fatal and developed epidemic proportions in England in the last four centuries, eventually requiring government intervention in the hope of controlling its spread. It was bacterial in origin and highly contagious by direct sexual contact. Its beginnings have been much debated, but syphilis seems to have been brought to Europe from America by Columbus's sailors returning in 1493, quickly spreading through Italy and France. Its name derives from a Latin poem by Fracastorus, written in 1530, telling the story of a shepherd named Syphilis, who so angered the gods that he was punished by this terrible affliction. Fracastorus considered that the disease would have serious consequences for the whole of Europe. The word syphilis was not used in the British lay press until 1913.

Syphilis was known in England from the early sixteenth century most often as the French Pox, but also as 'the Great Pox', 'le mal de Naples' and 'morbus gallicus', while the term 'clap' was in use by the 1580s. It was widely seen as a punishment from God for promiscuous behaviour, but self-inflicted, and so qualified medical practitioners generally did not treat sufferers, who had to seek attention from the assortment of quacks and charlatans that claimed to sell cures. The early sixteenth century in England saw an epidemic of syphilis lasting for some twenty-five years, until it became established as endemic, although having lost some of its severity by 1579 when William Clowes, a surgeon at St Bartholomew's Hospital, wrote his *Treatise Touching the Cure of the Disease called Morbus Gallicus*. Syphilis, unlike many other great infections of history, had an important congenital element, for it could afflict the unborn child with blindness and deafness, as well as causing mental and physical defects; it could also be passed on to the infant by breastfeeding. Gonorrhoea, on the other hand, was hard to diagnose, especially in women and, although rarely fatal, difficult to treat. It was a major cause of infertility in women and it was originally considered an initial stage of syphilis.

By the eighteenth century, cures for venereal infections were the most widely-advertised product in English newspapers, not always discreetly phrased. General acknowledgement of the disease may be seen in its many public references, in plays, novels and poems of the period, but above all in Hogarth's vivid depictions of both sufferers and quacks. His prints were very widely sold, often, as with *Industry and idleness*, hung in workplaces as bearing a moral tale. Thus in *The harlot's progress* (1734) we see Moll Hackabout, the country girl who became a prostitute, dying, 'poxed', at the age of twenty-three. In plate five, two quacks quarrel at her death bed, one of whom was John Misaubin, a venereal specialist, the other was Joshua ('Spot') Ward, inventor of the famous pill described in *Tom Jones* as 'flying at once to the particular part of the Body on which you desire to operate'. On the floor lies an advertisement for an 'Adonyne Necklace, the great Specific Remedy for the Secret Disease'. However, Hogarth also shows how a venereal infection plays a part in *Marriage-à-la-mode* (1745), for the unfaithful young nobleman is obliged to visit Monsr de la Pillule for treatment. He is accompanied by a young child and the consulting room in plate three is clearly meant to be that of Sir Samuel Garth, the poet-physician and author of 'The Dispensary'. Even when Hogarth shows the marriage contract being signed, the young Viscount Squanderfield is depicted with a patch hiding a venereal sore on his neck and the child's presence in the dispensary suggests that he was using her as a cure for his infection, for it was a widely-held belief at the time that sexual intercourse with a virgin would cure a man of syphilis. His young daughter is later seen wearing a leg-iron and with a sore on her cheek. In private papers, diaries and letters, writers also express fear of syphilis and accounts of their treatments. Thus William Hickey, noting his symptoms of the 'baneful disease' and his 'venereal taints', took Velno's Syrup, but eventually was treated by two leading London surgeons; Robert Adair gave him a course of salivation and mercury that lasted a month. The incorrigible James Boswell regarded an attack as 'merely the chance of war' in London in the 1760s and became infected repeatedly during his time there, perhaps not surprisingly, as he noted eleven encounters with prostitutes during nineteen weeks in 1763, only twice using a condom, although in January of that year he had been treated for his 'strong infection' by the surgeon, Andrew Douglas. Lord Byron suffered several venereal infections in his short life, one in February 1808, when he was treated by a London practitioner and wrote of it to his friend, Hobhouse:

> I am buried in an abyss of Sensuality, I have renounced *hazard* however, but I am given to Harlots, and live in a state of Concubinage. I am at this moment under a course of restoration by Pearson's prescription, for a debility occasioned by too frequent Connection [sexual intercourse]. Pearson sayeth, I have done sufficient with[in] these last ten days, to undermine my Constitution.

Six months later, he was buying a quack remedy for his symptoms.

Although mercury was the standard medical treatment for syphilis, it was acknowledged as dangerous, both immediately and long-term, and in fact it helped to dry up the superficial symptoms of the skin lesions, rather than conquer the infection. Guiacum, a herbal remedy based on bark and recommended by Fracastorus two hundred years earlier, was also widely used and, although ineffectual, it was at least harmless. Many sufferers thus bought the variety of patent medicines on sale in the Georgian sexual economy, all widely advertised and available. Such preparations became increasingly lucrative, with Lisbon Diet Drink, for example, costing 10s. 6d. a bottle; two bottles a day were required by the patient and one man claimed to have spent £300 on the mixture. One of the best-selling eighteenth-century nostrums for syphilis was Vegetable Balsam, made from sublimate of mercury, gum arabic, honey and syrup. It was produced by Nathaniel Godbold, originally a gingerbread baker, who made a profit of

£10,000 a year for the first decade after launching it. He bought Westwood Place, a fine country house near Godalming in 1790 for £30,000 and, on his death in 1799, a tablet in the parish church tactfully commemorated him as the 'inventor of that admirable medicine for consumptions and asthmas, the Vegetable Balsam'.

While syphilis remained a secret disease for individuals, it was already noted by authority, if only by barring sufferers from general hospitals. However, in 1747 the Lock Hospital was opened in a house in Grosvenor Place, London, a charitable venture specifically for venereal patients. It claimed that of the 695 patients admitted in its first two years, 646 were cured; about ten patients a year died while in residence. No patients were readmitted after discharge, so that the hospital could not be seen to be encouraging immorality. By 1784 it contained forty beds, including separate wards for women and infants; married women were noted as such on admission. To encourage moral reform a small chapel was added in 1762. Famous London actors were active patrons of the Lock Hospital, including David Garrick and Samuel Foote; Handel gave a benefit concert performance that raised £78 for the hospital's funds in 1753 and increasing numbers of Non-Conformists became its supporters. A refuge for prostitutes discharged as cured was added with William Wilberforce's help in 1787. At this period medical opinion, including John Hunter, still thought that gonorrhoea was simply an early stage of syphilis, rather than a lesser, non-fatal separate infection and the differences were not confirmed until as late as 1879.

Syphilis was essentially an urban disease, especially where there were army garrisons or naval stations that attracted prostitutes, but it was also common in London and the main cities. There were strikingly different attitudes to venereal infections between the eighteenth and nineteenth centuries, largely reflecting contemporary attitudes to sexuality generally, rakish and exuberant in Georgian England, maternal and serious in the Victorian era. However, the nineteenth century acknowledged the public health problems associated with venereal disease and provincial Lock Hospitals were built in Newcastle (1813), Manchester (1819), Liverpool (1834), Leeds (1842), Bristol (1870) and Brighton (1881), while many workhouses opened venereal wards. In the 1860s the sad case of Lady Mordaunt (see Chapter 6), when her new-born child suffered from an ophthalmic condition that appeared to be of venereal origin, indicates the powerful hold that such infections had on both popular and medical thought. Ibsen's Ghosts is only one example of how hereditary syphilis could be depicted in contemporary literature.

Government intervention occurred in 1864 when the Contagious Diseases Act was passed, to apply only to naval and garrison towns, requiring prostitutes to be compulsorily medically examined, staying in a Lock Hospital for between three and six months if they were found to be infected. However, five years later Josephine Butler founded an association, with support from such eminent campaigners as Florence Nightingale and Harriet Martineau, to have the Act repealed, arguing that it punished only prostitutes, not their clients. The struggle took some time, for in 1873 a Royal Commission and in 1882 a Select Committee of the House of Commons had reported in favour of the Act, which was not repealed until 1886.

The invention of an effective test for syphilis in 1906 by August Wasserman, followed by the development of arsenical Salvarsan 606, the 'magic bullet', by Paul Ehrlich four years later to replace the traditional mercurial therapy, made a cure for syphilis possible. Although Salvarsan was not devoid of risks for the patient, especially in its early stages, it was in practice a rational and scientific treatment, extensively used until the coming of penicillin and antibiotics. The Government's concern at rising figures for syphilis on the eve of the First World War resulted in a Royal Commission, which did not issue its report until 1916. This estimated that some 10 per cent of the urban population was infected with syphilis and more with gonorrhoea. The report did not refer to self-treatment by chemical disinfectants to reduce infection after sexual contact for fear of seeming to encourage immorality and condoms were not mentioned.

More positively, it recommended that local authorities should provide free diagnosis and treatment in clinics to reduce numbers carrying the disease, protecting patients' anonymity, encourage health education and add the subject to the curriculum of medical students. Advertisements for remedies were to be banned and the report essentially concentrated on treating VD rather than preventing its spread. VD clinics, often attached to existing hospitals, were established a year later and they remained the most general way of treating patients for forty years. Some hospitals would not participate because they would thus be 'condoning vice' and the VD centres would be outside the control of the traditional hospital governors. Some GPs were pleased to be able to pass patients on to the clinics. Centres opened in the London area in January 1917 and by the end of the year there were 113 clinics that had seen over 29,000 new cases. By 1920 the number had increased to 190 centres treating 105,185 patients and expenditure rose from £116,000 in 1917–18 to £287,000 in 1919–20. Shortage of practitioners to staff the clinics was a major problem and a number of ex-army medical officers were appointed. The proportion of women who attended the clinics was relatively few and women's hospitals did not take part in the scheme. However, as VD was not a notifiable disease, there are no really reliable statistics for the period, but it is clear that cases of syphilis fell throughout the 1920s and 1930s, although gonorrhoea numbers continued to rise until the coming of sulphonamides in the late 1930s. There was also some medical opposition to free, self-referral clinics as a threat to practitioners' incomes and the growing specialty of venerology. There was widespread concern at the huge increase in venereal diseases noted amongst the troops in the First World War, with a total of 383,706 diagnosed as infected in the period from April 1917 to December 1919. At demobilisation it inevitably spread to the civilian population. The issue of condoms to protect troops from infections had helped to bring about greater social acceptance of contraception, although 'mechanical devices' were condemned by the church as encouraging promiscuity. The armed services, of course, could use medical controls not possible in civilian life and awareness of breaching civil liberties in trying to reduce VD was a constant problem to reformers. By the Second World War, however, greater emphasis was placed on publicity and education of the public at large, with notification of contacts and compulsory treatment.

The extreme social upheaval of both world wars, especially that of 1939–45, had produced 'war aphrodisia', with a noticeable relaxation in sexual behaviour, especially for women. By 1941 the national VD statistics had increased by 70 per cent in two years, with even higher figures in London and the great ports; Liverpool, for example, saw a four-fold growth in cases. With the coming of American troops to England from the spring of 1942, national VD figures reached epidemic levels. Publicity to warn everyone of the risks of venereal infections was instituted, some of it especially graphic (Figure 8.2), and notices about treatment and clinics were displayed in all public lavatories. In the same six-year period, more than a third of all the infants born were illegitimate; before 1939 there were 5.5 births in a thousand that were illegitimate, a figure which peaked at 16.1 per thousand in 1945. With the use of antibiotic therapy, by 1956 syphilis and gonorrhoea had been so effectively treated that some VD clinics were closing for lack of patients. However, new, penicillin-resistant strains developed and, when the use of condoms diminished in favour of the contraceptive pill in the 1960s, venereal infections once again became an acute social and medical problem.

Of all epidemics, only venereal infections were primarily the result of social attitudes and personal behaviour but, as with other very different afflictions, government intervention was eventually required. Whereas medical advances were able to control smallpox through inoculation and vaccination, the other great scourges of English society were ultimately conquered by better water and improved sanitation, that were part of a generally raised standard of living across two centuries. Raised levels of natural immunity and loss of virulence in causal organisms cannot, of course, be measured, but must have played a part in certain diseases in accounting for the enormous population growth that occurred in England between the mid-eighteenth and mid-twentieth centuries, as did improved medical skills and services generally in two hundred years.

The startling rapidity of the population growth in Victorian Britain was, in fact, the real problem for reformers and practitioners alike and its concentration in towns at the root of most problems. Engels, in contrasting urban and rural living, had noted that 'dirty habits do no great harm in the countryside where the population is scattered ... the dangerous situation which develops when such habits are practised among the crowded population of big cities, must arouse feelings of apprenhension and disgust'. This concentration can be seen clearly in comparing 1801 and 1911, two census years. In 1801 only London had a population of over 100,000 (11 per cent of the whole nation); by 1851 there were ten such towns (25 per cent) and in 1911 there were thirty-six, comprising nearly 44 per cent of the population. Contemporary reformers, however, stressed the

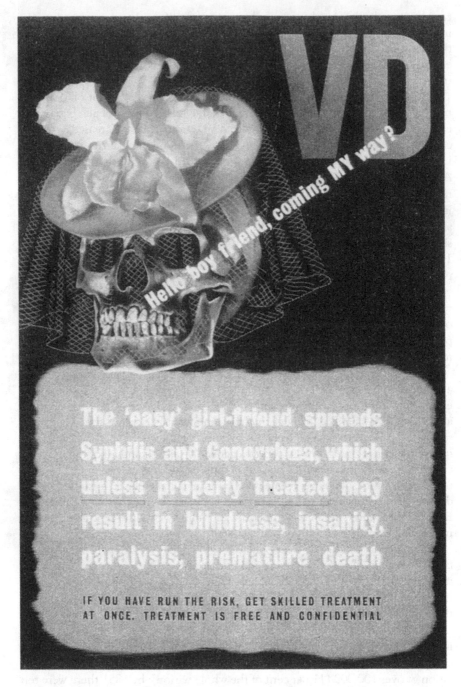

Figure 8.2 A poster warning of the dangers of VD. Designed by Reginald Mount, 1943–4. © Imperial War Museum.

differences in life expectancy between the social classes and from one location to another, an argument made by *The Lancet* on 5 August 1843. However, public health became a moral crusade and the basis for all other reforms, as well as a topic of comment in cartoons and of profit in medical advertisements.

As the death rate declined, especially in babies under the age of one, and as life expectancy rose from 40.2 in 1841 to 50.2 in 1911, there was a considerable degree of self-congratulation in official circles. However, conflicting views were raised by those such as Charles Masterman, who emphasised that the death rate had fallen due to better sanitation and 'increased medical skill', rather than to a better standard of living. The result was 'race decay', a sickly nation, vividly confirmed by the poor physical standards of recruits for the Boer War. Responses to this dilemma included the establishment of planned, model communities, such as Port Sunlight, near Liverpool, Bourneville, near Birmingham, or New Earswick, near York, all founded by grand philanthropic industrialists. There were also plans for slum clearance and garden cities, such as Letchworth. It was clear, however, from Rowntree's surveys in York, that the low levels of wages did not allow the poorest to keep themselves 'in a state of bare physical efficiency' and indeed at the outbreak of war in 1914 about a third of all wage-earners in the country were below Rowntree's poverty level. It is inescapable that although medical advances were made, life expectancy increased and public sanitation improved in over a century, the factors for good general health in the nation were many years away.

The Suttonian method of inoculation against smallpox, 1767

Richard Radcliffe to John James, senior, of Queen's College, Oxford

Dear James,

Your letter arrived at the proper time, and gave me a pleasure greater than usual. I was sorry however to hear, that mine had had such an effect upon my sister. I thought it might possibly occasion a surprise, but I never dreamt of its being attended with serious consequences. Inoculation has been practised in this country so much and with so great success, that it seems to have lost all it's terrors. I am willing to flatter myself, that I was not presumptuous or confident upon the occasion; though certain it is, that I was never more happy and cheerful in any part of my life. On Sunday, July 12, I received my instructions from Mr. Sutton; by which I was ordered to abstain from butter, cheese, spices, animal food of every kind, and from all vinous, spiritous, and malt liquors. Most luckily he does not forbid the use of tobacco, so that I indulged myself freely in my old custom, and drank my health in water, whey, milk well-skimmed or lemonade. On the same Sunday evening at bed time, I took a paper of his powders, supposed to be in preparation for the mercury, and in quantity not exceeding a good large pinch of snuff. The next morning I had the pleasure of swallowing about an ounce of Glaubar salts, and I dare say you will vastly rejoice to hear that they operated very briskly and plentifully. These powders and salts were repeated twice afterwards, resting two or three days between each dose. Being thus reduced and prepared I set out with six of my neighbours for Newark on Tuesday July the 21st. The doctor attended us instantly, and performed the operation upon us, which was done by dipping the point of his lancet in a pustule of one of his patients, and lightly piercing the outer skin in two different places on each arm, a little above the elbow. No blood was drawn, nor was the puncture hardly perceptible, so that there was no occasion for any plaister or bandage. On Wednesday we had the curiosity to examine our arms, and could perceive little red spots at the places of incision, exactly resembling a flea-bite. These spots continued to inflame every day and ripened at last into fine pustules, and then died away with the rest. On Thursday the doctor came again, and after due inspection, pronounced that we had all received the infection. This piece of intelligence pleased me most wonderfully, as it had been a matter or dispute among my friends, whether or no I had had the distemper. On Friday I was ordered to eat a little meat, and on Saturday to drink a little ale; an indulgence not allowed to any one else in the company. On Sunday I had, or fancied I had, a little touch of the head-ach; which, fortunately, was all the illness that fell to my share. On Monday evening or Tuesday morning an eruption appeared on that part of my body, which gentlemen of the birch are often indulged with a sight of; and this, with the pustules at the places of incision, was all I had to shew for my money. I am however assured by Mr. Sutton, and two other sensible and experienced gentlemen, that I have had the distemper very effectually, and that I never had it before. From that time I was allowed to eat, drink, and live as I pleased; and after paying the doctor five guineas, and expending about four pounds upon other occasions, I returned to Colsterworth the Tuesday following, with great satisfaction of mind, and (I trust) with a proper gratitude to the Great Dispenser of all things. My companions escaped wonderfully well, though not quite in the favourable manner that I did. Seventy people have been inoculated in this parish by a common country apothecary, all of whom have happily recovered, and none of them have suffered any thing worth speaking of.

Margaret Evans (ed.), *The Letters of Richard Radcliffe and John James of Queen's College, Oxford, 1755–83*, Oxford Historical Society, Oxford, 1888, pp. 25–7

Deaths in cholera epidemics in England, 1831–1866

County	1831	1849	1854	1866
Bedfordshire	40	72	61	22
Berkshire	52	148	49	3
Buckinghamshire	105	175	68	10
Cambridgeshire	208	269	271	7
Cheshire	111	653	141	391
Cornwall	308	835	24	21
Cumberland	702	419	35	32
Derbyshire	16	50	17	20
Devonshire	1901	2366	188	525
Dorset	19	122	45	6
Durham, County	850	1642	ns	352
Essex	38	580	513	471
Gloucestershire	932	1465	260	39
Hampshire	91	1245	130	417
Herefordshire	0	1	1	2
Hertfordshire	ns	323	97	9
Huntingdonshire	45	14	18	1
Kent	135	1208	1056	284
Lancashire	2835	8184	1775	2600
Leicestershire	5	8	14	3
Lincolnshire	80	372	134	48
London	5275	14,137	10,738	5596
Middlesex	62	406	380	51
Norfolk	232	223	381	15
Northamptonshire	0	141	152	7
Northumberland	1394	1417	ns	224
Nottinghamshire	352	137	80	12
Oxfordshire	219	117	183	4
Rutland	0	7	9	0
Shropshire	158	316	13	17
Somerset	142	923	21	68
Staffordshire	1870	2672	426	30
Suffolk	1	79	67	15
Surrey	0	255	252	82
Sussex	0	346	94	79
Warwickshire	188	293	89	15

County	1831	1849	1854	1866
Westmorland	68	1	1	1
Wiltshire	14	320	60	11
Worcestershire	579	432	103	36
Yorkshire, East Riding	507	2140	70	54
North Riding	47	47	84	21
West Riding	1416	4151	470	283

Figures based on analysis by Charles Creighton, A *History of Epidemics in Britain*, vol. 2
Note
ns = not stated

9

THE PHARMACEUTICAL INDUSTRY

The Druggist: His Business is to buy up, in large Quantities, all manner of uncompounded Drugs, both foreign and domestic; these he sells to the Apothecary, who compounds them: Yet, generally speaking, he compounds Drugs for Sale in his own Shop, like the Apothecary. The Druggist is not supposed to know any thing of the uses or Properties of Drugs: He only buys them as a Merchant, and disposes of them as a Commodity ... It is a very profitable Business ... their Returns sometimes *Cent. per Cent.* and seldom below Fifty.

R. Campbell, *The London Tradesman*, 1747, pp. 62–3

Although the pharmaceutical industry is a creation of the twentieth century, the apothecary's role in preparing medicines was crucial to the whole medical profession from the earliest period. However, Nicholas Culpeper is widely recognised as the author of the first pharmacopoeia written in English, and thus accessible to more readers, in contrast to earlier publications in Latin, such as the first *Pharmacopoeia Londonensis* of 1618. This volume was compiled by the London College of Physicians and described as well as classified the drugs and medications approved by the College. Culpeper's translation of this work in 1649, *A Physicall Directory*, went into two further editions in 1650 and 1677. In it, he classified over 1,100 simples and some 900 formulae for compounded medicines, over half of which were from ancient authors. This was an age of polypharmacy and over two hundred prescriptions contained ten or more ingredients each, while several had over fifty. The remarkable 'Antidotus magnus Mathioli', powerful against both poisons and bubonic plague, was compounded from over 130 substances. A number of medicines were made from animals, many also used in folk medicine, including grasshoppers, ants, swallows, lizards and vipers, little removed from *Macbeth*'s witches' brew. Of the thirty-five *animalia* given by Culpeper, many remained in the *Pharmacopoeia* until 1746, while three were still used into the twentieth century, cantharides, cochineal and leeches, the last still of value in modern microsurgery techniques. Culpeper's most popular work, however, was his herbal, *The English Physician Enlarged* (1653), written in English, with a strong astrological content and selling at a modest price.

161

The eighteenth century saw the development of a range of medications, many widely sold, such as Ormskirk Medicine, for example. Some were named after their inventors, not all of whom were empirics by any means; James's Powder, Kennedy's Lisbon Diet Drink and Morison's Paste were highly profitable products all devised by medical practitioners. The eighteenth and nineteenth centuries, however, were the heyday of quack medicines, heavily advertised, particularly in the press, widely available and some relatively expensive, usually a first step in self-treatment before a medical practitioner was consulted and paid. In the same period many factors were contributing to a lowered death-rate and increased population, including a raised standard of living and an improved environment, as well as such medical advances as inoculation/vaccination and better institutional health care in the form of hospitals and dispensaries. Professional medical education had also expanded the curricula taught and subjects on which students were examined.

However, drug production and distribution had changed little over the centuries. Large-scale drug wholesalers and importers traded in all important English towns, wealthy men who often held office as aldermen, mayors or sheriffs. As Campbell had noted, the druggist's was a very profitable trade, requiring between £500 and £2,000 to set up in business because of the large stock that had to be bought, held and distributed, some of it perishable. By the last decade of the eighteenth century, there were 463 druggists' firms in provincial England, including ten run by females, presumably widows or daughters of former traders continuing the family business. In the large towns druggists were well-represented in the community, with sixteen firms in Exeter and fifteen in both Bristol and Liverpool, for example, as well as in Manchester (13), Hull and Sheffield (10 each), while they were also prominent in Newcastle (9), Bath (8), Chester (8), Coventry (6) and Lincoln (6), all regional centres and most with county hospitals. The apothecaries, who were smaller retailers, trading in all but the remotest villages, bought supplies from the wholesale druggists and then sold medicines in small quantities direct to the public, as well as making up prescriptions and preparing their own nostrums for patients' symptoms, as many continued to do well into the twentieth century. Over-the-counter prescribing has been a feature of the pharmacist's skill for some three hundred years.

The increased specialisation of druggists can be clearly seen from the mid-eighteenth century onwards. Thus in 1767, when there were eleven druggists trading in Birmingham, four were also described as grocers and only one noted as a wholesale chemist. In that year, before the General Hospital opened, the medical personnel of Birmingham consisted of three physicians and twenty surgeon-apothecaries. By 1811 there were eighteen firms (two in partnerships and two run by women) and as early as 1818 one had a laboratory on the edge of the town. By 1850, however, with a five-fold increase in all practitioners there, there were nineteen manufacturing chemists, including six partnerships. Their typical prosperity may be judged by the fact that five wholesale chemists in Birmingham who died between 1834 and 1858 left sums between £14,000 and

£40,000. In the rest of the county, however, there was only one other manufacturing druggist, Wyleys of Coventry, a family firm founded in 1751 who continued to trade in the city for over two hundred years. As an indication of their prosperity, apprentices there regularly paid premiums of £100 to £200 for five or six years.

All the significant advances towards a modern pharmaceutical industry in the first half of the nineteenth century were made in Europe, for example, the work of Frederick Sertürner to isolate morphine from opium latex and of Joseph Pelletier to produce quinine from yellow bark. Europe also saw the invention of what were to become standard diagnostic tools, such as the stethoscope and the clinical thermometer.

By the middle of the nineteenth century manufacturing and wholesale chemists were trading in all parts of England, many with origins in an earlier age, such as Taylor, Brawne & Flood in Bedford (founded in 1780), Howards & Sons in Ilford (1797) or Bleasdale in York (1780). However, with the economic expansion of Victorian England, the majority of firms were founded in the middle decades of the nineteenth century, some still currently trading, either in their own name (for example, William Ransom of Hitchin, founded in 1845, and Smith & Nephew of Hull, founded in 1858) or as part of a multinational company. Thus Glaxo acquired Bradley & Bliss of Reading (founded in 1817), Thomas Morson of Enfield (1821) and Evans Medical of Leatherhead (1821), while Hoechst took over Arthur C. Cox of Barnstaple (1839) and AAH bought up other smaller firms, such as Ayrton, Saunders of Liverpool (1868) and Bleasdale of York.

The majority of early druggists predictably traded in London, as they had done for centuries. Thus Godfrey & Cooke, taken over by Savory & Moore in 1916, was founded in 1680 by a chemist who had formerly been Robert Boyle's assistant, while George Atkinson & Co. had been established in Aldersgate Street in 1654 and British Drug Houses included a wholesale firm dating back to 1650. Perhaps the most successful and certainly long-lasting of the London druggists was the partnership of Allen & Hanbury, established in 1715 at Old Plough Court by a Quaker, Silvanus Bevan, who was issuing a wholesale list before 1730. The patent medicine business was growing and in 1748 there were over two hundred preparations listed in *The Gentleman's Magazine*; by 1783 these were considered so reliable a source of extra revenue that the government established the Patent Medicine Stamp Act. In 1792 William Allen, aged only twenty-two, joined the firm, which was then trading with Europe and America, and married Charlotte Hanbury. At the turn of the century, the firm had a factory at Plaistow and a laboratory at Plough Court, where they took orders from mines and factories for chemical analysis. The firm was strictly disciplined; they were the first to use angular bottles for poisons, for example. Plough Court was extensively rebuilt in the mid-nineteenth century, expanding the retail activities and employing five dispensers and two shopmen. Their range included innovations such as photographic work and as general wholesalers they supplied retailers all over

England by the end of the century. The firm developed some well-known speciality products, for example, refined cod-liver oil, produced at the new Bethnal Green factory, malt extract as an infant food made by vacuum process and, its most famous creation, blackcurrant throat sweets, for which the name 'pastilles' was coined, using a special sugar-coating process unique to Allen & Hanbury. From the late eighteenth century the firm was making surgeons' instruments, a trade which continued into the twentieth century, with a new factory in 1940 and retail premises at Wigmore Street, London. Allen & Hanbury were one of only three English firms to manufacture insulin and also set up a pilot plant at Ware to produce penicillin. In 1958 they were taken over by Glaxo Ltd.

Originally, the early druggists ran essentially personal enterprises, often finding success through their own individual prescriptions. For example, Arthur H. Cox of Exeter in 1854 patented a pearl coating for pills that made them less unpleasant to swallow and Kay Brothers of Stockport manufactured a best-selling compound of essence of linseed; Beecham's pills, with the advertising slogan 'worth a guinea a box', were so successful a product that a new factory was built for their manufacture in 1876. As a public display of success, Thomas Holloway, a substantial London vendor of patent medicines, endowed Royal Holloway College (1879–87), 'the most ebullient building in the Home Counties' and built the Holloway Sanatorium at Virginia Water, which opened in 1884. The druggist business was highly competitive, even in the early days, and Henry Hodder of Bristol, founded in 1846, sold patent medicines at reduced prices, claiming to be the first 'cash chemist' in the country. A unique service was provided in London by John Bell & Croydon, founded by a Quaker in 1798, in their Wigmore Street shop in London, which remained open twenty-four hours a day and for 365 days a year from 1912 until 1966.

In the later nineteenth century in the provinces the most substantial firm was undoubtedly Boots of Nottingham. Jesse Boot took over the family business in Goosegate, Nottingham, in 1877 and changed virtually all aspects of wholesale and retail pharmacy. Whereas apprenticeship to a druggist had always involved high premiums, open only to boys from prosperous families, Jesse Boot took no premiums and paid his apprentices a weekly wage of 10s., thus allowing boys from a modest social background to become qualified. These youths were obviously destined to be the dispensers of the future rather than the capital-risking manufacturing druggists. Boots was to become the best-known supplier of patent and prescription medicines in England. In 1884 a branch was opened in Sheffield and by 1893, with thirty-three stores, Boots was the largest chemist's chain in the country, having become Boots Pure Drug Company Ltd in 1888. The retail chain consisted of 250 outlets by the turn of the century. The firm appointed its first welfare officer in 1911. In the First World War Boots set up a Research and Fine Chemicals Department to produce chemicals that had formerly been imported, for example, aspirin from Germany, and also manufactured box respirators against gas attacks. In the Second World War the firm produced large quantities of saccharin (to replace rationed sugar) and chloramine for water sterilisation.

Boots set up the largest surface culture plant in the world to produce penicillin, while a fermentation penicillin plant was a post-war development by Glaxo.

However, the architects of modern drug manufacture in England are generally considered to be the firm of Burroughs Wellcome, founded by two American pharmacists when they arrived in England in 1880. Silas Burroughs, who died in 1895, was essentially the salesman and traveller, while Wellcome was the inventor and practical innovator. Henry Wellcome had special machinery made that would manufacture a tablet of precise dosage, which became increasingly important with the development of new and powerful drugs; in 1884 he coined the word 'tabloid' for his new invention. Gelatine-coated capsules were a further innovation. He established one of the first research laboratories at Beckenham in 1894 to produce diphtheria antiserum and, under the direction of Henry Dale, also carried out research on ergot and digoxin. In 1923, within a year of its discovery in Canada, the firm began large-scale manufacture of insulin, the first made in Britain. During the First World War Wellcome had produced quantities of tetanus antitoxins, anti-gas gangrene sera and typhoid vaccines for the Western Front. In 1932 the Wellcome Institute opened in London for research into tropical diseases and to house the huge collection of historical medical artefacts, papers and books that Wellcome had amassed. He was knighted in 1932 and died four years later. An important modern innovation was analytical control throughout the manufacturing process and in 1954 Wellcome introduced a system of recording adverse reactions to any of their drugs. The thalidomide tragedy of 1959–61, in which some 12,000 babies worldwide were born with severe physical defects as a result of Distillers' drug to cure morning sickness in pregnancy, undoubtedly caused wider acceptance of such caution and the Wellcome system later became obligatory under the Committee of Safety of Medicines. The Company had become a worldwide enterprise and recent work has been done on interferon, acyclovir, antihistamines and an AIDS vaccine. Henry Wellcome loved catch-phrases such as 'Products of Quality' and 'Weapons of Precision' but his personal and professional philosophy was the pursuit of excellence; five Nobel Prize winners were employed by the firm.

In terms of drug innovation the nineteenth century can truly be said to be Germany's, especially when linked to such vital new diagnostic tools as microscopes, making possible the study of histology, linking anatomy and physiology, and where the laboratory predominated over the hospital. In addition, victory against France in 1870 undoubtedly brought a feeling of confidence in Germany's economy, encouraging industrial innovations. This was especially so in German efforts to synthesise drugs, since nature or a difficult international situation could unpredictably make a particular plant unavailable and stop the supply of a particular drug. These powerful new products, alkaloids, including morphine, digoxin, cocaine and quinine, could now be made with consistent quality, purity and strength and became a main feature of medical prescribing. The nineteenth century also saw preparations sold, some still widely available, for which new uses have recently been found, for example, aspirin in preventing heart attacks. Aspirin, however, has mid-eighteenth-century origins in the bark of the white willow used as an analgesic in folk medicine until commercially produced by Bayer and patented in 1899. It soon had universal sales and has been called the 'Drug of the Century'. In Britain, drug research was considerably impeded by the anti-vivisection movement, with Queen Victoria's support, and the 1876 Cruelty to Animals Act permitted only licensed medical practitioners to carry out vivisection.

A growing sense of professionalism among British wholesale druggists led to the formation of their own trade organisations. The Association of the British Pharmaceutical Industry was founded in London in 1891, originally known as the Drug Club, to ensure that products of the highest quality were readily available. By 1980 there were 154 manufacturing companies who were members of ABPI. Because this organisation was felt to reflect the interests of manufacturers rather than of wholesalers, in 1902 a rival group, the Northern Wholesale Druggists' Association, was formed, gradually extending its membership across other areas; the Association was dissolved in 1966.

In contrast to this development of scientific drugs, an enormous range of non-prescribed preparations continued to be sold to all social classes in all periods and it has been estimated that the British public bought more pills per capita than any other European nation in the nineteenth century, when some £2m. a year was spent on advertising these 'quack' products. However, even in the early 1800s the Stamp Acts of 1804 and 1812 produced considerable revenue for the government and later in the century some £3m. a year was raised in duty paid on these sales. There was, predictably perhaps, disapproval from the medical profession at this obvious high level of self-treatment and in the years 1868–1909 there were no fewer than six Acts of Parliament passed to control the sales of patent medicines, the Pharmacy Acts (1868–9), the Sale of Food and Drugs Acts (1875, 1899), the Merchandise Act (1887), the Indecent Advertisements Act (1889) and the Poisons and Pharmacy Act (1908). Although advertisements for quack remedies were common in the eighteenth-century press, by Victoria's reign, as general literacy improved, numbers of newpapers and magazines grew, so that the whole advertising 'industry' was able to promote consumer products as never before.

In response to medical disquiet that such cures were ineffectual or harmful and also reduced professional incomes, the BMA produced two surveys, *Secret Remedies – what they cost and what they contain* in 1909 and 1912 and a Select Committee was set up to investigate the whole question of patent medicines. Its *Report* was published in 1914, a thousand pages long based on the evidence of forty-two witnesses, eleven of them physicians, largely condemning 'this system of quackery'. The main problem for the Committee was that there was no definite line separating beneficial drugs from quack remedies and thirty such cures were included in the published *British Pharmacopoeia*, although this was administered by the medical profession from 1858. Certainly these remedies contributed to the 'medicalisation' of life in England and were particularly directed at such Victorian ailments as neurasthenia, 'sick headache' and 'loss of vigour'. However, patent medicines slowly moved closer to legitimate ones, so that aspirin, introduced in 1899, rapidly became the most popular drug in England and contemporary writers as different as Engels, Shaw, Conrad and George Eliot disapprovingly noted the trend to greater consumption of such preparations.

Although patent medicines continued to be sold in large quantities, the coming of the Health Insurance Act in 1911 brought considerable profits to the drug industry, with a dramatic increase in prescriptions as medical benefits became available to the working population. The outbreak of war in 1914 demonstrated how far the pharmaceutical industry was dominated by Germany, as British companies had distributed drugs but undertaken relatively little research into new products. Drug prices rose immediately in 1914, so that bromides rose from 1s. 6d. a pound to 10s., and some commodities were unavailable. The government forbade the export of fine chemicals and German subsidiaries in Britain were confiscated. The British firms pooled their information and set up the Medical Research Committee, which, for example, tested the British Salvarsan substitutes made by Burroughs Wellcome and May & Baker.

Local small chemists, however, continued to provide a substantial range of medication to the general public. Medical historians have long debated to what extent, if at all, medicine had any noticeable effects on the health of the nation, recently concluding that public health measures were more important and that improvements in health predated such major advances as immunisation, sulphonamides and antibiotics. In the last decades of the twentieth century chemotherapy and antibiotics, linked to surgical innovations, have been responsible for greater control of illness, with more emphasis on prevention (such as drugs to lower blood pressure), screening techniques and general health education. However, the great reduction in infant mortality and the control of childhood diseases has been perhaps the most significant factor of all in the nation's health, and in this area of medicine the drug industry has played an important part.

Specimen of the Price Book

Acacia Gum, the new name in the Pharmacopoeia of 1809, for **Gum Arabic.**

Hankey, 5s. 6d. – 5s. 6d. 3/j. *Drawer No. 1, East Corner.*

Tyrrel, 4s. 6d. old name GUMMI ARABICUM.

White, from 20d. New name, (Pharmacop. 1809) ACACIA GUMMI

—— **Powdered,** 6d. & 8d. 3/ *Spece Bottle, No. 1, second shelf,*

Hankey, 3s. 8d. *front.*

—— 4s. – 5s. 6d.

Jackson & Manley, PULVIS GUMMI ACACIÆ, or ARABICI.
4s. – 4s. 6d. to 5s. 6d.

William Chamberlaine, *Tyrocinium Medicum,* 1819, p. 144

Cash price list, W. B. & H. Holmes, Faversham, patent medicines, 1936

	s. d.
Abbey's Salt per bot.	3 0
Allcock's Porus Plasters	1 3
" Corn Shields	1 3
Allen and Hanbury's Perfected Cod Liver Oil	1s. 6d. and 2 6
" " " Tasteless Castor Oil	1s. 3d. and 2 3
" " " Bynin	2s. 9d. and 5 0
" " " Bynol	2s. and 3 6
Allenbury's Food, No. 1 and No. 2	2s. 1d. and 4 0
" " No. 3	1s. 3d., 2s. 6d. and 6 3
" " Diet	2s. 1d. and 4 0
" " Milk Cocoa	2s. and 3 6
" " Rusks	2s. 3d. and 4 6
Angier's Emulsion	3s. and 5 0
Aspro per pkt.	6d. and 1 3
Beeham's Patent Pills	1s. 3d. and 3 0
Beecham's Cough	1s. 3d. and 3 0
Beetham's Lait Larola	1s. 6d. and 2 6
Benbow's Dog Mixture	2 6
Benger's Food	2s. 3d. and 4 0
Benzine	7½d. and 10½d
Bile Beans	1 3
Bishop's Citrate of Magnesia	1s. 4d. and 2 6

Privately owned

10

MEDICINE AND WAR

We are McIndoe's Army
We are his Guinea Pigs,
With dermatomes and pedicles,
Glass eyes, false teeth and wigs.
And when we get our discharge
We'll shout with all our might
'Per ardua ad Astra'
We'd rather drink than fight.

John Hunter runs the gasworks,
Ross Tilley wields the knife,
And if you are not careful
They'll have your flaming life.
So Guinea Pigs, stand ready
For all your surgeons' calls,
And if their hands aren't steady
They'll whip off both your balls.

First two verses of *The Guinea Pig Anthem*, Anon., *c*. 1940

At any period when battles were fought, on land or at sea, medical attention was essential for the wounded and Hippocrates had advised 'He who wishes to be a surgeon should go to war'. However, certain characteristics applied to naval and military medicine that were absent from civilian practice, for patients, healthy young men, were forced to do as the surgeons decreed and there were a great number of patients with medical conditions all to be attended at the same time, immediately and in emergency conditions. A war situation provided dramatic wounds to be treated, frequently far from home and with the surgeons having to extemporise. As wars had to be won for reasons of national prestige, trade and empire, there was considerable political value to healthy fighting men who could secure victory and medical facilities were thus crucial. The desperate state of demobilised soldiers and sailors at the end of a war can be seen all over England in the accounts of parish constables, who regularly disbursed small sums, often 6d. each, to disbanded men carrying a government pass that enabled them to return home in peacetime without being arrested as vagrants.

As early as the sixteenth and seventeenth centuries practical naval and army surgeons, such as John Woodall and Richard Wiseman, wrote treatises on their experiences of attending the wounded, for which the English Civil War provided considerable scope. Certainly by this period, as guns and cannon replaced swords and arrows, there were greater demands on surgeons to treat far more serious gaping wounds. As a charitable venture, the Royal Hospital for Seamen was designed by Christopher Wren at Greenwich in the years 1682–92 and, with ceilings by Sir James Thornhill, was grander than many palaces. There was also a growing need, as the navy supporting British colonialism expanded in the early eighteenth century, for many more young surgeons, as the career of James Yonge of Plymouth exemplifies. After his apprenticeship, Yonge was ship's surgeon on voyages to Newfoundland and was captured by the Dutch before setting up in practice in Plymouth, where he was master to eleven apprentices, with whom he took premiums of between £40 and £90 in the years 1672–1703. In 1713 the British fleet comprised 247 vessels, each of which had a surgeon and his mate on board and such practitioners' experiences were graphically described by Tobias Smollett, himself a former ship's surgeon, in *Roderick Random* (1748). By 1783, there were 390 surgeons serving in the navy, as well as those attached to dock-yards such as Chatham, Deptford and Sheerness.

However, in spite of ships surgeons' activities, naval death rates were extremely high, largely from scurvy, which virtually decimated Anson's crew in his circumnavigation of the globe in 1740–44, when 16 per cent of his 1,955 men died from fevers and dysentery but 50.9 per cent (997 men) from scurvy. So many deaths in such a well-publicised achievement undoubtedly helped James Lind to press his claims for vitamin C treatment to prevent this scourge among sailors. His *Treaty on Scurvy* (1753) went into three editions; it was followed by a controlled trial on HMS *Salisbury*, Lind's own ship, a year later and the therapy of raw lemon juice was so successful that in Cook's voyage of 1770 there was only one death from scurvy. The general issue of lemon juice in the navy after six weeks at sea on salt rations from 1795 was certainly a factor in Britain's successes in the Napoleonic War, enabling British ships to remain longer at sea without constantly taking on fresh food supplies to prevent scurvy, essential in the blockade strategy of Admirals St Vincent, Cornwallis and Nelson. In 1853 the Admiralty changed to lime juice as a source of vitamin C, but this was less effective and scurvy reappeared: both Scott and Shackleton later suffered from the disease. Lind commented on vitamin C deficiency in the Seven Years' War that:

> The number of seamen in time of war who die by shipwreck, capture, famine, fire and sword are but inconsiderable in respect of such as are destroyed by the ship diseases and the usual maladies of intemperate climes.

In fact, 133,708 men died from disease or deserted, while only 512 were killed in action and it was not until 1921 that Frederick Gowland Hopkins presented his research on the importance of vitamins in nutrition.

At the same time that conditions at sea were improving, two great naval hospitals were being built on the south coast at Haslar and at Plymouth. The first naval hospital in fact had been established at Greenwich and handed over to the navy in 1694 (completed in 1728) and there were British naval hospitals founded overseas at important strategic points, for example, at Jamaica (1704), Minorca (1711) and Gibraltar (1746). However, in the war with Spain of 1739–40, the situation alarmed the government when 15,868 sick and wounded were landed from the fleet, most of them at Gosport and Plymouth. The Admiralty decided that it would be more economical to care for these men in institutions owned and run by the navy rather than paying for their care in various hospitals and at rented houses and inns when necessary. The Admiralty commissioned a 'strong, durable, plain building' at Haslar, near Gosport from Theodore Jacobsen, architect of the London Foundling Hospital. Work began at Haslar in 1746 and the hospital was completely finished in 1761, the biggest hospital and the largest brick building in Britain. It had 1,884 beds and its wards were spacious, measuring 60 feet by 24, some of which were specifically for those suffering from smallpox, consumption, dysentery and scurvy, as well as cells for lunatics. The Royal Naval Hospital at Plymouth (1758–62) could take 1,200 patients in sixty wards with similar special units. John Howard noted in 1784 that the Plymouth ward blocks were detached 'for the purpose of admitting freer circulation of air, as also of classing the several disorders in such manner, as may best prevent the spread of contagion'. Certainly Plymouth's death rate, lower than that of Haslar, confirmed the success of the design.

The medical staff were naval personnel and lived on the site in separate accommodation. Haslar had two physicians, Lind and his son, each paid £200 a year, as well as two surgeons (£150), with ten assistant surgeons, two visiting apothecaries and a dispenser (£100 each), who had eleven assistants. There was also the dockyard surgeon in Portsmouth, who was paid £100 a year and a contribution from each man of 2d. a month to his salary. At Plymouth there were fewer medical staff, one physician, one surgeon, two assistants, a dispenser and an assistant, but they were paid the same rates as at Haslar. The long-established Royal Hospital at Greenwich had the same number of medical staff as at Plymouth. Smaller new hospitals, each with three hundred beds, were later built at Deal (c. 1795) and Great Yarmouth (1809–11) during the Napoleonic Wars and one at Chatham with 252 beds in fourteen-bed wards in 1827–8. After the Crimean War, a new naval hospital was built in 1858 on the site of the Royal Marine Barracks at Woolwich, one of the first designed on the pavilion plan, with 273 beds, including wards for infectious patients.

Although the Royal Hospital at Chelsea, set in thirty-six acres, was designed by Christopher Wren as a 'Hospital of Maymed Soldiers' in 1682, military hospitals as such did not exist at this early period. However, medical care of soldiers changed dramatically from the eighteenth century onwards, a period of almost constant warfare for Britain. The eighteenth century saw the raising of county militia forces, consisting of men aged from eighteen to forty-five, with only clerics excused because of their occupation, as were apprentices and the disabled. The militia was required to fight only on the mainland, but freed the professional standing army to travel overseas to defend Britain's substantial colonies. All county militias had their own surgeons who served only when called out to join the unit; for this they were paid 4s. a day, but an Act of 1802 required that they be appointed in peacetime as well as when the regiment was active. A major health problem for militia regiments seemed to occur when they were stationed far from their home county and exposed to new infections. Thus in 1779 when the South Lincolnshire militia was stationed at Poole, they caught typhus from the crew of a captured French ship anchored in the harbour. Militia camps were usually retained until late in the summer when the weather began to deteriorate. Militia surgeons were given a medicine chest by the army's Apothecary General and an allowance of £7 10s. a month for a hospital in the camp. Medicines were paid for by weekly stoppages out of the soldiers' pay until 1783, but after 1792 a capitation scheme was devised for paying surgeons. In the last years of the eighteenth century when war was at its height, regiments demanded more surgeons from the War Office and surgeons required more regular salaries. The larger regiments also began to appoint assistants to the regimental surgeon as his work increased. Some surgeons gained extra salary by inoculating militia men; the Sussex regiment was inoculated at the expense of the Duke of Richmond in 1779, for example. As well as the 168 part-time surgeons, however, in 1783 the army in Britain had a full-time complement of nineteen physicians, fifty-four surgeons and thirty-one apothecaries, in addition to a few garrison surgeons (as at Woolwich and Berwick) and a small number of men on half-pay. Some also had distinguished careers in civilian practice; for example, Sir Clifton Wintringham, FRS, Physician General to the Forces and later royal physician, had attended the wounded in Flanders in 1743, while John Hunter, who had served in the Belle Isle campaign in 1761, later became Surgeon General to the Land Forces and Inspector General of Hospitals.

Army hospital facilities, however, were minimal and temporary, with hired rooms being used in a regiment's own area or tented accommodation (known as 'flying' hospitals) near the battlefield when needed. The first purpose-built army hospital in 1745 was at Berwick-upon-Tweed as part of the large barracks there, for some forty patients. During the War of the Austrian Succession (1742–8) it was agreed that hospitals should be regarded as neutral in the conflict. After this war had ended, the Physician General to His Majesty's Forces Overseas, Sir John Pringle, wrote his *Observations on the Diseases of the Army in Camp and Garrison* (1752) demanding cleaner accommodation, smaller groups of patients, a minimum of 36 square feet per hospital patient and praising the virtues of fresh air for the sick, a discovery he had made when noting the beneficial effects of a broken window as he inspected a particular hospital. In this war there was a death rate of 7.9 per cent and three of the serving eight physicians died. In the same period, John Ranby, an active force in securing the surgeons' professional separation from the barbers, wrote his *Method of Treating Gunshot Wounds* (1744), based on his personal experiences and preferring primary amputation, a view not shared by John Hunter. After the battle of Dettingen only thirty out of three hundred amputations were recorded as 'cured', a success rate which must have partly accounted for the numbers of crippled beggars commonly noted on the streets of British cities.

However, the Seven Years' War (1756–63) saw improvements in medical services to the army. Pitt himself understood the importance of fit and healthy fighting men for the war and set out his criteria that recruits were 'to be none but able bodied men, free from rupture and every other distemper and impurity that may render them unfit for duty, not under 17 or above 40, five feet four inches and above'. A new post, that of Inspector of Regimental Infirmaries, was created at the outbreak of war, and Robert Adair was the first surgeon to be appointed, although hospital directors were still military rather than medical men. In addition, new barracks meant healthier troops and a better diet was introduced. Medical examination for new recruits also began, although not widely practised until 1790, and higher rates of pay for surgeons secured a better grade of entrant. Their pay was raised to £250 a year in 1764. The standards of military hospitals remained appalling, so that in 1764 Richard Brocklesby MD, later Physician to the Army, could write of the average army hospital:

> Most commonly the habitation hired for an infirmary has for some time been unoccupied, with the walls all damp, the boarded floors half rotten, and the roof in several places open above … I have seen such a cottage stuffed with 40, 50, or 60, nay with 70 or 80 poor soldiers all lying heel to head, so closely confined together with their own stinking cloathes, foul linen, etc., that it was enough to suffocate the patients as well as others who were obliged to approach them.

British colonies were considerably expanded at this period and came to include tropical locations such as Tobago and Senegal, where the death rate for European soldiers was extremely high. As a result of his experiences as a surgeon in the West Indies, John Hunter wrote *The Blood, Inflammation and Gun Shot Wounds* (posthumously published in 1794), based on what he had seen of the seven hundred soldiers killed and wounded in April 1761. In spite of the lessons that should have been learned from the Seven Years' War, nothing was done until the return of wounded men from the former American colonies led to the building of army hospitals by 1781 at Portsmouth (for sixty men), Chatham (sixty) and Carisbrooke, although no evidence of these institutions has survived. However, hospital facilities were available to individual soldiers through the existing county infirmaries, as at Birmingham, for example, where two or three serving men a year were admitted as emergencies in the decades before military hospitals opened.

The first purpose-built general hospitals for the military, however, were at Gosport in 1796 and at Plymouth and Walmer a year later. The largest of these with 362 beds was at Plymouth, sited opposite the great Royal Naval Hospital, whose plan it echoed. The hospital at Walmer was similar but smaller. In fact, the Army Board was divided in its views on the necessity of military hospitals in Britain and was still inclined to undertake conversions, as at Chelsea, where the York Hospital for five hundred was created from the Star and Garter inn, rather than the commitment of a new building. However, the return of troops from Egypt in 1801 with severe eye infections (trachoma) led to the army's establishing a specialist ophthalmic depot at Selsey, an innovation later to be copied in civilian medicine at Moorfields Eye Hospital (1804–5). The disease also occurred when British troops fought in other very hot locations, as in India, Malta and Buenos Aires, for example, and by 1810 there were 2,317 soldiers entered on the army pension list as blind. At the Selsey depot John Vetch, surgeon of the 52nd Regiment, treated over three thousand ophthalmic cases in the years 1806–12 and noted 58 per cent as 'cured'. A further innovation of this period was to begin protecting troops against smallpox and in 1801 two civilian practitioners travelled to Egypt to vaccinate all the men serving there under Lt Gen. Sir Ralph Abercromby.

The later period of the Napoleonic Wars saw many changes in medical provisions for the army. For his ten thousand men in the Peninsular War (1808–11) Wellington had a medical staff of nineteen, including two physicians, four surgeons, one apothecary and ten hospital 'mates'; he referred to them as 'the medical gentlemen'. There were still no orderlies recruited, and such tasks as stretcher-bearing were traditionally done by the regimental musicians. Hospitals were set up in Lisbon and other larger towns and Wellington unsuccessfully requested thirty more hospital 'mates', to combat not only battle wounds but also the fevers and dysentery of summer and the respiratory diseases of winter. As well as the hospitals, other local accommodation was being used, and one young Connaught Ranger gave a vivid description of the scene in the courtyard of a nobleman's house, where he:

> saw about two hundred wounded soldiers waiting to have their limbs amputated, while others were arriving every moment. It would be difficult to convey an idea of the frightful appearance of these men; they had been wounded on the 5th and this was the 7th; their limbs were swollen to an enormous size, and the smell from the gunshot wounds was dreadful ... as many of them were wounded in the head as well as in the limbs, the ghastly countenances of these poor fellows presented a dismal sight. The streams of gore which had trickled down their cheeks was quite hardened with the sun, and gave their faces a copper-coloured hue; their eyes were sunk and fixed, they resembled more a group of bronze figures than anything human.

He then described the activities of the surgeons, 'stripped to their shirts and bloody', using doors raised on barrels as temporary operating tables, 'to the right were arms and legs, flung here and there without distinction, and the ground was dyed with blood'. The scale of the problem was such that in 1811 alone there were 14,000 men in hospital in the Peninsula.

Large numbers of the men repatriated at the end of Wellington's peninsular campaign were suffering from typhus, but several British military hospitals had earlier been closed down to save money, although Haslar naval hospital took in many patients and civilian practitioners in the Portsmouth area attended others. When the battle of Waterloo took place, a substantial number of army surgeons already had considerable battlefield experience. Five British hospitals were established in Belgium, but losses were extremely high and in an area of some two square miles there were over 40,000 dead and wounded. As well as the 7,016 men wounded at Waterloo, there were 2,380 from the earlier battle of Quatre Bras; with the French casualties, some 15,000 beds were needed. The injured included the grandest military figures, such as Lord Raglan, who had an arm amputated, and Lord Uxbridge, who lost a leg. Sir Charles Bell, later Professor of Surgery at Edinburgh, who published *Dissertation on Gun-shot Wounds* (1814) wrote of operating for twelve hours a day there, when

> All the decencies of performing surgical operations were soon neglected; while I amputated one man's thigh there lay at one time thirteen all beseeching to be taken next. It was strange to feel my clothes stiff with blood and my arms powerless with the exertion of using my knife.

After Waterloo for the first time military surgeons became eligible for a grant of prize money; there were seventy-two out of a total of 206 serving on 15–18 June who benefitted. As a result of the Napoleonic Wars a new military general hospital was built at Fort Pitt near Chatham (1805–19) and began admitting patients in 1814; it was replaced by a larger version in 1823–4, with eight big wards each of twenty-seven beds, which, however, proved impossible to heat effectively. The last pre-Crimean military hospital to be built was at Portsmouth, with 279 beds, in about 1853.

The effects of the 'most unnecessary war in modern Europe', the Crimean, on British nursing are widely acknowledged, but the war also had far-reaching consequences for military medicine generally, including the design and provision of hospitals in Britain. As the country had been at peace for forty years, both the army and its medical services were distinctly unprepared for battle and the War Office hoped the army would employ the Peninsular style of living off the invaded land, using local transport and food supplies. The Black Sea area was wholly unknown to the War Office and three practitioners were sent there to assess the medical risks for the troops of diseases and climate. The risks were all too tragically to be recognised as fevers, including malaria, typhus and later cholera, with exceptionally severe winters for which existing British army uni-

175

forms were wholly inadequate. When war was declared on 27 March 1854 the army medical department had no orderlies or waggon drivers and had to rely on 370 pensioners as volunteers. All equipment, even the necessary 550 beds, had to be ordered and medicines arrived three months late. When the British force of 20,000 arrived in the Crimea in September 1854, their hospital at Scutari opened using Turkish medical supplies; there were 174 medical officers, one for every 144 men.

Lack of transport for casualties dominated everything and only twenty-four local carts were available for medical use. After the victorious battle of the Alma, there were 1,800 wounded to be evacuated onto ships to be taken to Scutari, which was three hundred miles or three to five days sailing from the Crimea. The Scutari hospital, formerly Turkish barracks, consisted of 1,086 beds, spread along some four miles of wards, with insanitary latrines and a burial ground immediately to the south of the hospital. However, medical considerations did not press heavily on military tactics, and Lord Raglan was quite prepared to engage in a campaign with not a single hospital bed nearer than Scutari, where 2,300 patients were admitted after the battle of Inkerman.

Shortages became widespread as the first winter drew near; fuel for cooking and forage for horses became equally scarce and scurvy appeared among the troops as food supplies were limited, for fresh vegetables had never been part of army rations. In some cases, shortages were simply the result of poor administration, so that there were stocks of winter clothing and blankets held in the purveyor's department but not issued to the soldiers or sent to the hospitals. A decision was taken to improve the situation at Scutari by employing female nurses and the Secretary for War, the Duke of Newcastle, explained this radical scheme:

> When we found the great complaints that were made, and which were conveyed to me, not merely by the public press, and by private letters, but by gentlemen who came over from Constantinople at the time, and who had recently visited the hospitals, we felt it our duty to take such steps as we could to remedy such a state of things, and we reverted to the proposal of nurses. The difficulty was to find any lady who was competent to undertake so great a task ...

When Florence Nightingale and her first thirty-eight nurses arrived at Scutari on 4 November 1854 and she realised the scale of the problem, she not only requested eighty more nurses but also three hundred scrubbing brushes, so unhygienic were the conditions she found; two thousand men had died in two months from hospital infections. As she later acknowledged, however, she did not address the most significant cause of hospital deaths, the abysmal sanitation at Scutari, where more men died following amputation than when the operation took place in the field. In the winter of 1854–5, when trench warfare produced frostbite, 34.8 per cent of the whole British army were in hospital. Her middle-aged nurses were relatively well paid at 12s. to 14s. a week and their duties consisted of dressing wounds and feeding the seriously ill, as well as reading and writing letters for their patients. Although short supplies remained a problem, one of Florence Nightingale's strengths was that she could contact Sidney Herbert direct at the War Office and report events at Scutari. Thus in January 1855 she wrote:

> I am a kind of general dealer in socks, shirts, knives and forks, wooden spoons, tin baths, tables and forms, cabbages and carrots, operating tables, towels and soap, small tooth combs, precipitate for destroying lice, scissors, bed pans, and stump pillows ...

She had, in fact, ample funds for buying whatever was needed, collected from subscribers in Britain and with the active help of *The Times,* in which William Russell's vivid and critical Crimean reports were published. Aberdeen's government was to fall in January 1855 as a result of mismanaging the war and improvements were made; for example, new equipment and 10,000 sets of suitable clothing were sent to the Crimea. It was recognised that an ambulance corps was needed and better facilities on hospital ships. A means of transporting the wounded, the Hospital Conveyance Corps, to carry stretchers and drive wagons, was formed in May 1854, renamed a year later as the Land Transport Corps. A Medical Staff Corps was formed by royal warrant in 1855, especially for hospital service, and was replaced by the Army Hospital Corps a year later. In March 1855 under the new government a Sanitary Commission was sent out to Scutari, including three practitioners, an engineer and three sanitary inspectors; Florence Nightingale wrote to Lord Shaftesbury that 'it was this Commission that saved the British army'.

Florence Nightingale was undeniably seen by the public as a heroine but, as she herself recognised, became hated in various medical circles. She constantly clashed with Sir John Hall, Principal Medical Officer, especially over his pronouncement forbidding the use of chloroform in wound amputations. However, by the middle of the war, it was used in 95 per cent of all amputations. Throughout the whole Crimean War, medical demands for supplies were resisted by the army boards. Control was divided between the medical and military officers, so that, for example, there was little or no military insistence on general hygiene among the soldiers and the medical department felt they were blamed for the high death rates in the war when better supplies and less bureaucracy would have saved many lives. In Britain the medical services were centred on Chatham, where the Crimean sick and wounded were sent on their return to England; a total of 9,544 men were invalided as a result of the war. In all, 16,000 British troops died of sickness, fewer than 2,600 were killed in battle and 1,800 died of their wounds. Among the dead were fifty-five medical personnel, including thirteen surgeons and eighteen assistant surgeons. A Royal Commission of 1857 enquired into the disaster that had been the Crimean War. Florence Nightingale came to believe that 'construction generates disease' and, with the support of William Farr, the first Registrar General, increasingly promoted the new sanitary theories, including writing articles on the subject for *The Builder*. As Fort Pitt facilities were clearly inadequate, in 1856 a new thousand-bed hospital for the army was opened by Queen Victoria at Netley, near Southampton Water, but criticised as not built on the pavilion plan. The first hospital to provide officers' wards, it later included the main army lunatic asylum. It was demolished in 1966 and only the chapel, dedicated to St Luke, has survived.

A Royal Commission in 1857 approved the new Hospital Corps, insisting that its members should all be literate, not then a normal requirement for NCOs and privates. In 1865 a medical school for officers was founded at Fort Pitt, three years later it moved to Netley and then to Millbank, London in 1902. In 1875 the Royal Army Medical Corps established its depot at Aldershot and its royal warrant was issued on 23 June 1898. The RAMC was awarded a striking number of Victoria Crosses, including three in the Crimea, in the various wars of the later nineteenth century and in both World Wars.

The Boer War (1899–1902), however, indicated that the military medical services were sadly under-manned. At its beginning, the RAMC sent 850 medical officers to South Africa, with ten hospitals; by the end of the conflict, there were 8,500 Corps members and 21,000 beds in this distant country. This was a particularly difficult war for the British army, including its medical services, far from base and supplies, in an unhealthy climate, with considerable critical publicity of the whole campaign at home. In fact, typhoid killed more men (13,000) than the Boers (8,000) and the war brought reforms that were to be crucial when the European conflict broke out in 1914. Thus in the First World War typhoid was very rare, even at Gallipoli, with the introduction of mass inoculation and a death rate of only 2 per cent, compared with 10 per cent in South Africa. In the Boer War field hospitals were used for the first time and, as the rifle was the main weapon in South Africa, considerable medical experience was gained there of small calibre bullet wounds, to be critical in 1914–18. It was also discovered that 40 per cent of the volunteers for the Boer War in 1899 were medically unfit. In Manchester alone only a tenth of the 12,000 volunteers in 1901 were accepted; overall four in every ten men were rejected for rickets, skin diseases, and chronic bronchitis, most with teeth too rotten to chew properly. These rejected recruits were in fact no better than the poor specimens noted in Birmingham in the 1840s and political alarm led to the establishment of the Physical Deterioration Committee in 1904, with a particular interest in child health.

The First World War presented the thousand officers of the RAMC with a whole range of new enemy weapons and hazards, including shrapnel, grenades, machine guns, high explosive shells and gas, while completely novel methods of warfare, such as tanks and aircraft, brought new injuries and wounds. In this war, for the first time, deaths from wounds exceeded those from sickness and shell-fire injuries were far worse than those from bullets. Unprecedentedly long trench warfare in the heavily infected soil of the Western Front brought its own risks, including trench foot, trench fever and trench nephritis. However, there were medical innovations to respond to these hazards, for example, skin transplants, blood transfusions in the field, irrigation for wound cleansing and new antiseptics, such as flavine and dichloramine, as well as a range of inoculations against tetanus, gas gangrene and typhoid.

The problem of sheer numbers of casualties was one the RAMC had never faced before; thus after the attack on Loos on 25 September 1915 there were 37,000 wounded requiring treatment. In Britain in 1914 there were only 7,000 beds for the sick and wounded; by 1918 this number had increased to 364,000, many in temporary and hutted hospitals, with civilian buildings, such as large private houses (Woburn Abbey and Cliveden), pressed into use. As the war dragged on, the numbers of wounded returning to Britain from the Western Front swelled; there were 42,000 in May 1915, 108,000 in October 1916 and 93,000 in April 1918. Transport was a constant problem and, as well as horse and motor ambulances, sixty-three trains and sixty-six ships were converted to carry casualties. Perhaps the greatest medical challenge of the Western Front, however, was Germany's use of poisonous chlorine gas, which began on 22 April 1915 at Ypres. Lethal phosgene and mustard gases followed. Initially, the British army had no gas masks, relying on pads soaked in urine for some protection, but the War Office set up two research laboratories and gas masks were made in three months; a total of twenty-seven million were eventually produced. The scale of the problem is illustrated in the 195,000 British gas casualties, 9,000 of which were fatal. There was no effective treatment for extensive lung damage, while chlorine gas caused blindness, as hauntingly depicted in H. R. Mackey's painting, *The RAMC on active service* (Figure 10.1).

Warfare in other parts of the world brought specific medical problems for the army. Compounding the administrative muddle in the Middle East, of the total force of 163,000 sent to Gallipoli, only 40,000 were killed or missing, while 115,000 were casualties, particularly from a dysentery epidemic, so important that it became the subject of a Medical Research Committee enquiry. Sufferers were sent from Gallipoli on hospital ships to Malta to convalesce. Water-borne diseases, combined with the lack of supplies, were the greatest hazard in Mesopotamia, where 820,000 men were non-battle casualties and 85,000 were killed or wounded. There the medical conditions were vividly depicted by Stanley Spencer in his nineteen paintings at the Sandham Memorial Chapel in Burghclere. Spencer had himself spent part of the war in Bristol as an orderly and later served in Macedonia. The highest death rate of all was in German East Africa, where diseases accounted for over thirty times the number of men wounded by the enemy, described by General Smuts as 'a campaign against nature, in which climate, geography and disease fought more effectively against us than the well trained forces of the enemy'.

A significant aspect of medicine in the First World War were the opportunities for qualified women practitioners to work in areas that were formerly exclusively for men. By January 1917 more than half the male British medical profession had been called up and in the summer of that year there were 'great and unforeseen

179

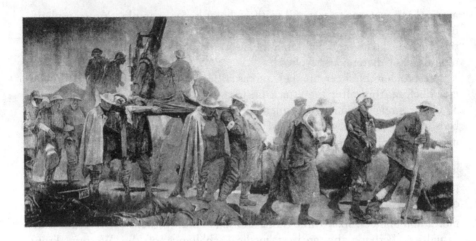

Figure 10.1 The RAMC on active service by H. R. Mackey. © The Wellcome Institute Library, London.

casualties in the commissioned ranks of the RAMC'. Civilian posts for female practitioners occurred in hospitals and attached to munitions factories but, as the War Office initially would not accept women in a war zone, they joined Allied medical teams. Although the War Office was finally obliged to use their services, women were never given commissions, but treated as civilians attached to the RAMC on short-term contracts, with uniforms provided only in June 1918. Commissioned rank was not achieved until the Second World War. Such strictures did not, however, stop several independent women's groups from medical service in the Middle East and on the Western Front, invariably self-funded, they had professional roles, especially as surgeons, that they were denied in Britain. A rare example of achievement in Britain was that Florence Stoney ran the X-ray unit at Fulham Military Hospital throughout the war, responsible for some 15,000 cases.

The unprecedented demands placed on the medical services in the 1914–18 war brought great advances in therapies and equipment, some of relevance later in civilian practice. Notable improvements were made in orthopaedic surgery, the beginnings of plastic surgery and the growth of radiology, with fourteen mobile and 528 fixed X-ray units, and the development of casualty clearing stations for the Western Front. The problems of mental health, especially in shell-shocked men, exemplified by Siegfried Sassoon and Wilfred Owen, came to be more sympathetically considered and many sufferers were repatriated. Although a similar condition known as 'traumatic neurasthenia' had been recognised as early as the 1860s, the first English description of shell shock was published in *The Lancet* in 1915, when hypnosis was noted as a treatment, and its editorial two years later called for greater attention to psychiatric medicine. In the first month of the war, the President of the Psycho-Medical Society had written to the War Office urging that a special hospital for such cases would be needed and the first one was opened in January 1915. In the period 1916–18 a programme was begun at Maghull Hospital, Lancashire, which trained sixty-five medical officers in psychiatry. It was not, however, until the unprecedently fierce fighting of the Somme in 1916 that there was a vast increase in shell shock cases. At this point there was concern that the diagnosis was being misused, with serious future demands for army pensions, and articles on the subject in both the *BMJ* and the *Journal of the RAMC* were blocked at the request of the Director General of the RAMC. However, there was widespread hostility to the diagnosis of shell shock throughout the British army and it was cited as a reason in the cases of some of the three hundred British soldiers executed for desertion or cowardice. The description 'shell shock' was largely avoided after 1917, especially as it was diagnosed in men who had never been near the front line, although it became the second greatest medical problem, after wounds, in the First World War. It was considered to be largely a condition suffered by the non-commissioned ranks and in the case of Siegfried Sassoon, who had won an MC for courage, the medical board tried to prove him insane rather than guilty of wilful refusal to fight. In 1917 he was sent to Craiglockhart War Hospital near Edinburgh, an institution for shell-shocked officers. As an interesting comparison, in 1939–45, some 40 per cent of all discharges from the army were for mental disorders.

Civilian life in the First World War was far less affected in practical terms than it was to be in 1939–45, when air raids were a major cause of civilian casualties. However, there were acknowledged occupational health risks in several essential war-time industries, especially munitions, for a hitherto domestic workforce. To reduce daytime drinking by the factory workers, new licensing laws were introduced in 1915, obliging pubs to close for four hours from 2 pm, whereas they had formerly been open all day, as well as reducing the strength of both beer and spirits. Official figures show that, during the war, beer and spirit consumption fell by 63 and 52 per cent respectively. Problems with food supplies, although never as severe as in the Second World War, brought about nutrition research, including the work of Gowland Hopkins in the inter-war years. When conscription was introduced for the first time in 1915, the government was concerned to discover that nearly half the men medically examined were only grades III ('with marked physical disabilities' fit only for clerical work) and IV ('totally and permanently unfit for military service'). Such discoveries were to have significant effects on welfare reforms in the inter-war years. However, civilian health was more disastrously affected at the end of the war by the great influenza pandemic than by enemy action in the four years of war. The long-term effects of the war were considerable, not least in the 1.3m receiving service pensions in 1918, some 9 per cent of whom suffered from heart disease.

In spite of its name, the First World War was not truly worldwide, for there were certain areas where no fighting took place and where British troops were not in action, particularly the Far East, while the civilian population in mainland Britain was largely safe from attack. However, in the Second World War, the Far East became a significant war zone, with malaria a particular health hazard in the Burma campaign, and the later rescue of survivors from Japanese prisoner of war camps a major task for the RAMC. North Africa was a completely new area for warfare and brought with it special health problems of climate and harsh physical conditions, where many techniques were improved of necessity, for example, resuscitation by intravenous fluids, with innovations such as packing a wound with sterile gauze or the Tobruk plaster (a Thomas splint incorporated in plaster of Paris). In this campaign, soldiers were provided with packets of sulphonamide powder to tip into a wound immediately and so reduce infection. The RAMC dealt with seven thousand casualties after the battle of El Alamein alone. Field surgical units were developed to provide forward surgical facilities close to the site of battle and an RAMC team formed part of the élite Long Range Desert Group.

Unlike the First World War, the Second World War saw virtually no fighting on the Western Front between the Dunkirk evacuation and the D-Day landings. However, certain other areas of conflict had particularly heavy casualties with unfamiliar terrain and very difficult conditions for medical care; after the four battles for Monte Cassino, for example, ambulance aircraft were needed to remove the very large numbers of wounded. Medical preparations for D-Day had been planned early in 1943, even to the provision of hyoscine for sea sickness and the modification of tank landing craft to carry three hundred wounded each. Extensive hygiene precautions included the issue of condoms to the troops. The Allies had 190 medical units in all and 1,154 RAMC personnel landed in Normandy in the first wave, as well as a field ambulance division with the 6th Airborne Division; 588 RAMC men were dropped at Arnhem by glider or parachute. The Corps was also involved in initially treating those released from the German labour and concentration camps, including Belsen. At the end of the war the RAMC's efforts were described by Field Marshal Montgomery in a message from Berlin as a 'contribution to victory ... beyond all calculation'.

Although the Royal Flying Corps had been formed in 1912, its duties initially were to cater for the requirements of the navy and the army, with no separate existence. An RAMC officer was attached to the Central Flying School on Salisbury Plain, although the RFC in France were not allocated their own medical officers until 1916. Research had already been carried out on mountain sickness and it was known that early balloonists lost consciousness at great heights, but no work was done in England on the medical hazards of flying, although research was being undertaken in France. Indeed, the attitude of the RAMC was that 'there are no special medical problems of flying' and pilots were treated basically for wounds and crashes; the stress of flying was not to be medically recognised for some time. However, eye tests and ear, nose and throat examinations for the many would-be pilots were slowly introduced, known as the Flack Tests, in 1917, essential when it was costing the War Office £2,000 to train a flier. The whole service expanded in numbers from 160,000 in these early years to 291,000 officers and men by 1918. The first published piece of research on aviation medicine, *The Value of Oxygen at Relatively Low Altitudes* (1917), by C. B. Heald, an RFC medical officer, appeared at this time. Since both the army and the navy wished to control the medical arm of the embryonic flying corps, it was decided that an independent service should be created. A Medical Flight was formed at Stanmore Aerodrome, near Hendon, which led to basic improvements, for example, in the design of flying suits and in the supply of oxygen at altitude. *The Lancet* was a firm supporter of aviation medicine and published seven articles and editorials on the topic during 1918. Progress was made when the RFC set up its own small hospital and research laboratory at Wimereux in the last phase of the war.

In Britain, RFC patients were sent to existing army and navy hospitals but in 1918, when the Royal Air Force came into being, a purpose-built station hospital was opened at Hendon, with three wards to take forty-two patients, including twelve females. The first general RAF hospital was at Halton Camp in Buckinghamshire, hutted accommodation that was made permanent in 1924-7 as Princess Mary's RAF Hospital. Among the greatest differences in conflict between two world wars was the emphasis in 1939-45 on air power as a means of victory and of prime significance in aviation medicine was the work of Harold Gillies and Archibald McIndoe, his cousin, both New Zealanders, at the Queen Victoria Hospital, East Grinstead. As early as 1920 Gillies had published *Plastic Surgery of the Face* based on his work in the First World War, when he set up a clinic at Aldershot. In 1916 after the Battle of the Somme alone he treated some two thousand patients needing facial surgery. Gillies was joined at East Grinstead by McIndoe as consultant plastic surgeon to the RAF in 1939 and after the Battle of Britain they treated about four thousand injured airmen with horrific burns, mostly from aviation fuel. At East Grinstead they promoted rehabilitation as well as what Gillies called 'reconstructive surgery', requiring an average of twelve operations for each patient. The men from ward three, a Nissen hut at the Queen Victoria Hospital, all survivors of blazing aircraft, formed themselves into the Guinea Pig Club; there were 644 members at the end of the war. Most of them had flown Hurricanes, since survival from a burning Spitfire, with its eighty-five gallon fuel tank, was rare. Other air force hospitals were built during the war, at Ely (1939-40), and at Wroughton (1939-42), as well as station hospitals. The RAF hospitals treated 70 per cent of air force personnel, the rest attending army and navy establishments.

Although the Second World War was essentially an event involving all British civilians, medical services in the 1930s were local and fragmented. However, the prospect of war obliged the authorities to establish the Emergency Medical Services, which were based on regional administration and a unified hospital service, critical for the later NHS, as well as national blood transfusion and ambulance services (see Chapter 11). The *blitzkreig* style of warfare used in Spain in 1936 had alerted the British government to devise some form of emergency service in the event of war, using the so-called 'Barcelona Ratio', that for every one tonne bomb dropped there would be some seventy-two casualties. Preparations began in 1937 by creating base hospitals at a safe distance from the large cities, when it was realised that bed capacity would be sadly inadequate for the 290,000 casualties anticipated from air raids. In preparation for war and following a hospital survey carried out early in 1938, an extra 50,000 beds were made available by a process of 'clearance', moving elderly and mental patients to make way for air raid casualties. In addition, a variety of huts and buildings were requisitioned across the country to provide a further 40,000 beds if necessary. Demands on hospital beds were greatly increased after the evacuation of Dunkirk in May 1940, the date on which air raids also began, and again after the V1 and V2 German rocket raids in 1944. Bomb damage to hospitals was a major problem, as flying bombs hit a hundred British hospitals, seventy-six of them in London. The demand for civilian nurses was acute in 1939, although recruitment was good into the military nursing ranks, and the government tried to increase numbers by visiting schools to persuade girls to volunteer for training. In 1939 there were some 60,000 trained nurses in institutions in England and Wales; by 1946 this number had increased by 8,000. As early as 1937 the BMA had begun to compile a list of general practitioners willing to work under emergency conditions in the event of war breaking out; 90 per cent of the medical profession entered their names on this list. By 1939 some 2,500 had enrolled for the Emergency Medical Services (EMS), some part-time. From April 1940 male practitioners up to the age of forty-one could be called up for military service, leaving a large proportion of senior hospital consultants for civilian work. Eight months later a Committee of Enquiry on Medical Personnel was set up to report on the situation. The EMS amalgamated with the NHS in July 1948.

In 1939–45 propaganda and new media methods, linked with psychological warfare, flourished, especially contrasted with the simple cartoon level of propaganda in earlier conflicts. Keeping up civilian morale was considered essential, especially as air raids became increasingly severe, and neither bread nor beer was ever rationed. The many civilians who remembered war only twenty years earlier must have seen great differences between the two World Wars. In 1939–45 women were vitally involved in the armed services, whereas in 1914–18 their most active roles had been in nursing, particularly overseas, including the VAD, the Queen Alexandra Royal Army Nursing Corps (QARANC) and the First Aid Nursing Yeomanry (FANY), as well as in making munitions in Britain and taking over male employment while the war lasted. Because of the risk of bombing raids, in 1939 nearly 1.5m mothers and children were speedily evacuated from such industrial centres as London, Liverpool and Newcastle to the safer rural areas, an exercise known as Operation Pied Piper. For the first time prosperous country dwellers came into direct contact with the urban poor, but recent research has suggested that the arrangements were far from perfect and within four months only a quarter of the evacuees remained in the receiving areas. As gas attacks were feared, gasmasks were distributed to all civilians, including very young children, who had cartoon characters decorating theirs. German bombing of civilian targets, especially city centres, was expected and a network of public air-raid shelters was organised. Their use also brought minor health problems: as many citizens from different backgrounds were all crowded together, infections such as sarcoptic mange and infestations persisted. The substantial numbers of civilian casualties severely strained hospital resources and medical facilities generally as younger practitioners left civilian life for the services. New responses such as large-scale blood transfusion arrangements across Britain were fairly quickly in place and government rationing secured adequately nutritious food supplies for all, since importing became virtually impossible as German U-boats attacked British merchant shipping. Different and healthier eating habits were forced on the nation, with less animal protein and more fibre in the diet. Infant mortality declined and the average age of death from natural causes went up during the war period. Social problems such as increased illegitimacy and rates of venereal disease were a further burden on the medical services of a country at war. Special diets were available for pregnant women and young children, while the whole population was urged to become self-sufficient by growing more of their own food, and indeed food production doubled from pre-war figures. In spite of the Second World War lasting for six years the general health of the civilian population was good and the diets of poorer people were better than they had been in the 1930s. The roots of the National Health Service may be said to lie in the lessons of the Second World War.

Of the wounds received in the actions of April 1782 by Sir Gilbert Blane

It frequently happens that men bleed to death before assistance can be procured, or lose so much blood as not to be able to go through an operation. In order to prevent this, it has been proposed and on some occasions practised to make each man carry about him a garter, or piece of rope-yarn in order to bind up a limb in case of profuse bleeding. If it should be objected that this, from its solemnity, may be apt to intimidate common men, officers at least should make use of some such precaution, especially as many of them, and those of the highest rank, are stationed on the quarter deck, which is one of the most exposed situations, and far removed from the cockpit, where the surgeon and his assistants are placed. This was the cause of the death of Captain Bayne, of the *Alfred*, who, having had his knee so shattered with a round shot, that it was necessary to amputate the limb, expired under the operation, in consequence of the weakness induced by the loss of blood in carrying him so far. As the Admiral [Rodney], on these occasions, allowed me the honour of being at his side, I carried in my pocket several tourniquets of a simple construction, in case accidents to any person on the quarterdeck should have required their use.

Christopher Lloyd (ed.), *The Health of Seamen*, The Navy Records Society, CVII, 1965, p.173

A nurse's diary, 1915, at Biyech on the Russian front

I was bandaging a young soldier, shot through the lung, when the first heavy shell fell. He was sitting up sideways against the wall, a wound the size of a small coin on his right breast and a wound big enough to put my hand into in his back. His right lung had been cruelly rent and his breath was coming out of the large back-wound in gurgling, bubbling sobs. The wounds had been quickly cleaned; the larger one filled with long swabs, a pad tightly bound over it, when an angry hiss was heard, grew louder and louder and then the explosion! The roar was deafening, the room shook and there were frightening noises of splintering, slicing masonry and of glass breaking and falling. A great silence followed, but the room continued to shake and tremble; or was it, perhaps, our own limbs? The soldier in front of me was shaking as with ague. 'Chemodan! [heavy shell]' he whispered hoarsely. I turned towards the table for a new roll of bandage. When I returned my patient had disappeared. In his half-bandaged condition he had run off, not caring for aught else and possessed with the one wild desire to escape to a safer place.

Florence Farmborough, *Nurse at the Russian Front* (1974), p.43

11

THE NATIONAL HEALTH
SERVICE

It will provide you with all medical, dental, and nursing care. Everyone – rich
or poor, man, woman or child – can use it or any part of it. There are no
charges, except for a few special items. There are no insurance qualifications.
But it is not a "charity". You are all paying for it, mainly as taxpayers, and it
will relieve your money worries in time of illness.

Ministry of Health leaflet, distributed to households, April 1948

The establishment of the National Health Service in Britain may be seen as a
direct outcome of the Second World War, when new and equal conditions were
promised to and expected by a victorious nation and when, driven by the
demands of war, medical skills had considerably advanced. Indeed, the
Emergency Medical Services had paved the way towards an integrated health
service, for war had forced medical services to cooperate as never before, removing many of the traditional barriers between hospitals, local authorities and
individual practitioners. However, free national health care had been a major
objective of the Labour party since 1934 and had even earlier antecedents in
the Royal Sanitary Commission of 1871, Sir John Simon's proposals of 1891 and
the Webbs' Minority Report in 1909 to the Poor Law Commission. The
Socialist Medical Association, founded in 1930 and affiliated to the Labour
Party a year later, had long favoured nationalised hospitals, health centres and
a state-funded salaried service. Certainly the coming of National Insurance in
1911 had made some of the population less dependent on the Poor Law in sickness, but its provisions essentially covered only those earning less than £160 a
year, aged sixteen to seventy, who were on a GP's 'panel' of patients; their
dependants were excluded. There were 19.2m panel patients by 1936, comprising 54 per cent of the adult British population. However, by 1938 plans had
been discussed either to expand the existing national health insurance schemes
to cover more of the population or develop the local authorities' existing services, ideas dismissed by their critics as utopian. By 1938–9, middle class patients
were spending 7–8 per cent of their income on medical care. All such plans
were inevitably halted by the outbreak of war. However, the coalition formed in

May 1940 brought into the government Labour politicians who were pledged to a free and comprehensive health service.

The Beveridge Report was published in November 1942, a month after the victory of El Alamein, strongly supported by Aneurin Bevan and Herbert Morrison but reluctantly accepted by Churchill, who, unwilling for anything to detract from the war effort, was opposed to all forms of social security and welfare. Attacking Beveridge's declared enemies, the five giants of Want, Ignorance, Disease, Squalor and Idleness, was unwelcome to the Treasury on the grounds of expense (the cost was estimated at £130m) and because they thought a welfare programme would undermine the work incentive. Beveridge proposed a flat rate for all contributors, benefits for everyone and a centrally-administered scheme; he aimed at 'security with freedom and responsibility'. He presumed a free national health service, full employment and family allowances. Even in the interwar years, local authorities had covered the costs of VD services, as well as employing health visitors, midwives and district nurses. They had also inherited the Victorian Poor Law infirmaries after 1929.

The hospital sector in fact was the most difficult aspect of planning the National Health Service. By the late 1930s many of the voluntary hospitals faced financial problems as charitable resources did not keep pace with increasingly costly treatments, in spite of support from hospital Saturday and Sunday Funds, and they were all sited in traditional centres of population. Until the EMS was formed, they were entirely separate from the public hospitals and from local authority services. It is clear that changes were brought about directly as a result of the war, removing established barriers from all the health care professions. The importance of the EMS was that it set up regional networks for treatment and introduced hospital staff to public work on a salaried basis, both important aspects of the new NHS, with a shift in emphasis from local to national, and with hospitals as central to the scheme. The EMS had also brought the middle class into direct contact, through voluntary work and as patients, with the poor facilities in many hospitals. War had made state intervention in civilian life, as in food rationing and evacuation, acceptable.

The attitude of the medical profession to any changes away from private practice was one of pessimism and, like the voluntary hospitals, they were unwilling to be swallowed up in a unified scheme as state employees, although even before the war the British Medical Association had published A General Medical Service for the Nation (1938) to consider the possibility. In the years 1936–8, the average practitioner's income was £950 a year, made up less from panel and more from private fee-paying patients, although the BMA was concerned that even then general practice was being eroded by expanding public health services and by hospital contributory schemes. However, as the war progressed, a widespread view seemed to grow that health should be a public priority. The Beveridge Committee on Social Insurance and Allied Services sat from June 1941 and, when it reported a year later, it called for

> A comprehensive national health service [that] will ensure that for every citizen there is available whatever medical treatment he requires in whatever form he requires it, domiciliary or institutional, general, specialist or consultant, and will ensure also the provision of dental, ophthalmic and surgical appliances, nursing and midwifery and rehabilitation after accidents.

However, remunerating medical practitioners was a major difficulty in establishing the NHS, for as well as income from private patients, capitation fees from friendly societies and the like, practitioners had always been able to buy and sell their practices and partnerships, with the goodwill attached, as well as equipment (and frequently premises) at valuation, just like any other business enterprise. Goodwill represented vitally important capital to the practitioner who moved or retired and was an asset, worth £2–3000 by the mid-1930s, to be sold on death. Medical relationships with the government had undoubtedly soured in 1941 when the National Health Insurance (NHI) level for panel patients was raised from an upper annual income of £250 to £420, thereby including many middle class patients from whom general practitioners had formerly received fees. The Treasury, meanwhile, was entirely opposed to medical salaries in any new scheme. In 1944 one GP wrote, 'We are fighting this bloodiest of all wars for freedom and this is not the time to put forward a scheme that will, in the short passage of time, take freedom away from the doctor and freedom and privacy from the patient'. A lengthy draft White Paper, keenly awaited, was prepared in January 1944, and the immediate reception was positive, a 'fresh stage in the course of domestic reconstruction'. Many Labour stalwarts felt it did not go far enough, especially Clement Attlee, who called it 'tentative and unhelpful'. However, the medical profession's reaction was lukewarm, wanting any changes to be effected slowly, and the government emphasised the provisional nature of all the proposals, hoping thus to secure the BMA's support. In the draft plan, friendly societies, for all their two centuries' existence, were given no role and mental health was hardly considered, although later included. At this point the debate had reached stalemate, the BMA insisting that such radical changes should wait until the war was over and a new government elected.

Labour withdrew from the coalition and came to power with an overall majority of 146 following a general election on 26 July 1945. Aneurin Bevan was made Minister of Health, at forty-seven the youngest member of the Cabinet, and the fourteenth man to hold the post, a political graveyard, since its creation in 1919. He was certainly an unconventional choice but quickly pushed through plans for a national health service, riding roughshod over many to do so. A miner's son who had left school at thirteen to go down the pit, he knew first-hand how the Medical Aid Societies of the Welsh coalfields and the NHI panel functioned; he was elected as an MP in 1929 for the safe Labour seat of Ebbw Vale. Within a month of becoming Minister of Health, Bevan had rejected all the former drafts and suggestions for national health schemes and put forward his own plan to be rid of 'silent suffering' in August 1945 with amazing speed. He steered the outline proposals through the Cabinet in October, the bill became law on 6 November 1945 and the NHS Act was passed in April 1946. The British public and the media warmly welcomed the plans and, although local authorities were unhappy at the proposed costs they would have to meet, the majority were Labour-controlled and so accepted what was so obviously and widely popular. The NHS came into full operation on time in 1948.

In the NHS, directly controlled by the Minister of Health, there was to be state intervention over where doctors practised, a new salary structure, the sale of goodwill was prohibited and health centres on the Scandinavian model were planned for the long term. The most dramatic change was that all hospitals were nationalised and were to be controlled through new regional authorities, except the thirty-six teaching hospitals, which were to be administered by boards of governors. A small number of pay beds for private patients were to be permitted in state hospitals and consultants of all specialisms were to receive the same fees within the NHS. General practitioners were to be paid £300 a year as a salary plus capitation fees for the number of patients on their lists. They resisted the salary element and wanted only capitation fees, a dispute in which Bevan gave way. Local authorities were to be responsible for domiciliary and child welfare services, local clinics and ambulances. The NHS thus became the third largest non-military organisation in the country (ranking after the British Transport Commission and the National Coal Board) with some 500,000 employees. Of these, 360,000 were employed in hospitals, 150,000 as nurses and midwives. In all these proposals Bevan would consult but not negotiate, although, having announced that the sale of practices was not allowed, he made arrangements for practitioners to be compensated financially for the loss of goodwill and £66m was set aside for this.

In these discussions, Bevan was seen as dictatorial, especially by the general practitioners, with whom relations were certainly strained. When the BMA had conducted a plebiscite among its members, of an 81 per cent poll, 54 per cent were against even continuing discussions. After Bevan had deliberately attacked the BMA in the House of Commons as 'politically poisoned' and 'raucous voiced', there were 48,814 practitioners against the NHS proposals and only 4,735 in favour. However, the widely-respected royal physician, Lord Moran, had intervened and secured a promise from Bevan that full-time salaried service should not be compulsory for practitioners and by May 1948 26 per cent of English GPs joined the NHS (36 per cent in Scotland and Wales) and two months later the list was almost full. By this time there were considerable numbers of practitioners being demobilised after wartime service; those over the age of forty-four returned to civilian life first. To many of the younger doctors the new proposals were attractive; they wished to enter civilian practice and cannot have welcomed the prospect of buying goodwill outright or purchasing a partnership share in an existing practice, frequently borrowing money to do so.

In launching the NHS country-wide publicity was employed in advance of the Appointed Day, 5 July 1948, exactly a hundred years after the first Public Health Act had been passed. Ministerial discussions began in February and Cabinet views differed on how best to introduce this radical scheme to the population. Herbert Morrison wished to promote the NHS as part of a larger plan for post-war reorganisation, but Bevan wanted publicity only for the health scheme. His view prevailed and a free leaflet was released in April to thirteen million households, its launch kept secret from the BMA. In fact, the free household leaflet, as with its contemporary, *The Highway Code*, was a favoured means of disseminating information for the new Labour government. Bevan thought the NHS leaflet 'the most powerful instrument in the armoury of publicity'. Films were used to spread the message further, including a ten minute cartoon, *Your Very Good Health*, and advertisements in the press declared 'This day makes history'. The Prime Minister, Clement Attlee, made a radio broadcast on the NHS to the nation at 9.15 pm on 4 July 1948. Six days later there were sixteen million new names of patients in England and Wales on the Executive Councils' lists, in addition to the 19.5m already there from the old NHI scheme.

Although estimates of costs had been made for the NHS, it was acknowledged in Bevan's circle that these were little more than fiction. There were really no accurate figures for the pre-war years on which to base predictions, but the annual budget for 1938 had been £16m. It was also widely believed that costs could be kept within limits and Bevan himself thought that, as free medical attention began to take effect, the nation's health would improve overall and in the long term the NHS would be less expensive to run as a low-cost preventative service. In the event, costs for 1948 exceeded the projected figure and increases had to be set for 1949–50, with £330m as the gross estimate. Concern was so great at having spent £10m over budget that in 1950 the NHS Cabinet Committee was set up to monitor running costs. It is clear that there had been no appreciation of the backlog of demand by patients, especially for dental and ophthalmic treatment, as free dentures, spectacles and even wigs were all well publicised. There was no yardstick against which to estimate for a wholly new enterprise and medical salaries in all areas were rising, although ministers thought that this particular difficulty would stabilise.

The greatest demands came from opticians (an increase of 460 per cent), to whom £3.5m had been allocated for the first year, whereas the first nine months of the scheme actually cost £15m. By 1951 cutbacks had been instituted and a charge was made for NHS spectacles. Dentistry costs, to be controlled by the Dental Estimates Board, calculated at less than £10m a year, were to be £41m in 1949 alone. When charges were introduced in 1951, dentistry costs were reduced by 66 per cent in two years. Other increased demands came from local authorities (300 per cent) and from the hospitals, which had needed extensive refurbishment and modernisation programmes, taking over half of the whole NHS budget. Thus teaching hospitals showed cost increases of 90 per cent but non-teaching hospitals of only 24 per cent. Not all other increases were rising so alarmingly (39 per cent from chemists, only 8 per cent from GPs). Bevan was convinced that savings could be made, but obviously not immediately. The Treasury decided to reduce hospitals' capital expenditure and for the first time the suggestion of in-patients contributing, if only to 'hotel' charges, was made, on this occasion by Stafford Cripps, the Chancellor of the Exchequer. One of his officials commented, 'In principle, I think a charge is right. I have never been able to see why people should get dentures and spectacles for nothing, any more than houses, food and clothing'.

Bevan's stance on the whole question of charges, on which he is widely believed to have resigned, was far from simple. Rather than accept charges for dental and ophthalmic treatments, which were not available to the poor before the NHS, he agreed to charges being levied on prescriptions, to bring in £10m a year, which he hoped would also end unnecessary prescribing, an argument emphasised by Attlee. The drug bill was rising remorselessly, from £18m in 1948–9 to £114m in 1963–4, not merely in numbers of prescriptions dispensed but in the range and costliness of actual drugs, so that pharmaceutical costs came to overtake the expense of general medical services. Bevan feared that NHS charges would lead to demands for higher old age pensions and that, if economies could not be made on health expenditure, cuts in the housing budget, a project dear to his heart, would be inevitable. He defended the prescription charge of 1s. per script, not per item, with the famous remark, 'I shudder to think at the ceaseless cascade of medicine which is pouring down British throats at the present time'. In fact, the average number of prescriptions per patient was 5.2 a year. He insisted that the prescription charge was only a short-term temporary measure, to be rescinded when funds permitted, whereas after his resignation he denied that he had ever intended to have prescription charges at all. As early as the summer of 1949 Stafford Cripps demanded a review of social service expenditure, although NHS charges were seen as politically very damaging, and on 3 April 1950 Bevan argued that 'the abandonment of a free and comprehensive health service would be a shock to our supporters and a grave disappointment to socialist opinion throughout the world'.

To soften resistance to the prescription charge, there were to be exempted categories of patients, those with war disability pensions (0.75m), those receiving National Assistance (0.75m) and old age pensioners (4.25m). These exclusions moreover would cost £4m and Bevan was firmly opposed to all exemptions. He managed, however, to endure the smallest share of government economies as the Budget was planned and insisted that, for such trivial savings, cuts would be politically harmful in the run-up to the General Election. Attlee agreed to defer a decision on the NHS cuts until after the country had voted. In fact, the NHS needed far more money spent on it than prescription charges would bring in and these were not implemented until 1952, under a Conservative government.

In the Budget for April 1951 Hugh Gaitskill demanded £40m saving on health costs, with a ceiling of £400m; as well as the shilling prescription charge, patients were to pay half the cost of dentures and £1 towards a pair of spectacles. Apart from NHS charges, income tax was raised by 6d. in the pound and purchase tax was doubled from 33 to 66 per cent. Bevan pressed for defence cuts, but to no avail, as the Korean War (1950–3) was in progress, and in addition the country was also suffering from a serious balance of payment problem and an increase in old age pensions. Aneurin Bevan resigned as Minister of Health on 27 April 1951, followed a day later by Harold Wilson. The Prime Minister, Clement Attlee, was in hospital at this crucial time. Bevan was made Minister of Labour and the Health post was removed from the Cabinet. The new Minister of Health was Hilary Marquand, formerly in the Ministry of Pensions, a great contrast to Bevan, described as 'dull' and 'no orator' in his obituary notice in *The Times* twenty years later. After a Conservative election victory on 25 October 1951, the new Minister of Health was Iain Macleod, a general practitioner's son. The new NHS, however, was effectively divided into three sectors: local authorities, the hospitals and primary care, of which only the second and third were to change significantly after 1948, for local authorities continued to control most of the services they had provided during the Second World War.

Hospitals

Although the war had necessitated cooperation between various branches in health care, the hospitals had retained their considerable independence, particularly the great old teaching hospitals, essentially the élite part of the service. The former Poor Law infirmaries, largely controlled by local authorities, were far more amenable to NHS changes. In 1948, there were 1,143 former voluntary hospitals (with 90,000 beds) and 1,545 municipal ones (390,000 beds) and in December 1945 the Cabinet were told that £97m a year would be needed to run the service and £3m to modernise it. By 1948, however, this estimate had increased to £121m and actual expenditure continued to rise; £345m was needed in 1955–6 and spending on hospitals accounted for 57 per cent of all the NHS budget. The reasons for this enormous share of the NHS budget were obvious; virtually all the buildings were old and had not been repaired, or had even been bombed, during the war. Regional surveys of hospitals were undertaken, all with depressing observations:

> the bulk of the hospitals in the region are out of date, their arrangements do not conform to modern needs and they are often too small with no possibility of expansion. Out-patient departments at general hospitals are especially poor, inconvenient and cramped.

England was divided into fourteen Regional Hospital Boards, the most notable innovation of the NHS, most comprising three or more counties. Thus, the South Western RHB covered Cornwall, Devon, Somerset, Gloucestershire and part of Wiltshire. Some boundaries were difficult to draw, as, for example, between Liverpool and Manchester RHBs, and each region had between three and four million as its population. Some areas were noted as particularly deprived, with poor resources allocated to them, and in 1947 East Anglia and Sheffield came in this category, with low staff/patient ratios as well as fewer and less well-qualified consultants. In addition, fourteen New Towns had been created, none of which had a hospital, although these were to be built in Welwyn and Harlow, for example. Poor Law institutions needed such modern facilities as X-ray units and pathology laboratories. In 1943 the philosophy of rationalisation was to be:

> An improvement in staffing and equipment, extensive adaptation of existing facilities, the provision of new services and accommodation, and substitution of a unified plan on a regional basis developed from considerations of geography, population, transport, communications, existing hospital accommodation and, where possible, a teaching centre.

Traditionally at the top of the hospital pyramid were the old-established teaching hospitals, thirty-six in England and Wales, but with a high proportion, twelve, in London. The key institution of each region was to be a teaching hospital. The teaching hospitals bridled at the uniformity of the new system, while the non-teaching establishments equally resented the more generous staffing levels and other advantages enjoyed by the London teaching hospitals. Many teaching hospitals, of course, had private resources of their own, often from their very earliest days, that produced income and thus independence from much government interference; some teaching hospitals refused to work with the regional services. Staff costs were rising as more medical and administrative personnel were recruited and as salaries increased, although hospitals were regularly accused of being over-staffed. There was certainly a 15 per cent increase in hospital staffing levels in the years 1949–52, especially in the administrative and clerical sections, and as early as March 1949 Cripps had asked Bevan to control hospital staff numbers, although some months earlier he had already agreed to make £50m cuts in hospital expenditure at the request of the Treasury. More economies were to follow in 1950 and waiting lists of patients seeking hospital admission were forming everywhere. A further problem in the 1950s was that all the existing hospitals were on old inner-city sites, from which the residential population had moved, although Addenbrooke's (at Cambridge) and the Radcliffe Infirmary (Oxford), both major teaching hospitals founded in the eighteenth century, eventually moved to new locations in the 1960s. The first new NHS hospitals to be built were at Swindon, the Princess Margaret general hospital, begun in 1957, and the Welwyn/Hatfield Queen Elizabeth II district hospital, opened in 1965.

Undoubtedly a major difficulty for Bevan in dealing with the hospitals in the early years of the NHS was the role and strength of the consultants within the medical profession. Initially he was convinced that they would participate if offered sufficiently high remuneration and become full-time salaried employees of the NHS. However, the consultants could look back to two centuries of private practice and of virtual independence in the hospitals and were strongly opposed to giving up their traditional status and privileges within the new scheme. Problems included the distinctive career pattern within the hospital service, requiring at least seven years to reach even junior consultant grade, as well as the unpopularity of certain essential specialisms (psychiatry, anaesthetics, pathology, radiology) and the difficulties of recruiting in some less favoured geographical areas. Numbers of overseas practitioners, the majority from the Commonwealth, were engaged to fill some of these vacancies. However, Bevan finally agreed that consultants should be allowed to hold part-time appointments under the NHS, still treating their private patients and receiving fees, and with access to pay beds in NHS hospitals. The majority of consultants chose this path. Bevan did not succeed by 'stuffing their mouths with gold' as he had anticipated, although consultants had financial security through their state salaries, while the distinction awards system provided additional income for meritorious service. The idea came from Lord Moran, who presided over the awards committee, and was welcomed by the profession's leaders. Awards ranged from £500 to £2,500, although details were never disclosed before 1958. The nationalisation and regionalisation of the hospital service was undoubtedly the most original feature of Bevan's reforms. This was especially so at a time when great professional changes were occurring in hospital medicine (so that, for example, chest surgery was more occupied with lung cancer than, as formerly, with tuberculosis) and also as social pressures virtually institutionalised childbirth out of the home.

Mental hospitals

As early as 1926, when the Royal Commission on Lunacy prepared its report, it was assumed that mental health services would develop separately from general health facilities and indeed asylums were omitted both from war-time surveys and from the early drafts on hospital reorganisation. In 1946 there were 147,000 mental patients in institutional care, as well as 53,000 'mental deficiency patients', 47,000 in the community and some 100,000 still in the community needing care (about 347,000 in all), as well as over 20,000 workhouse inhabitants in this category. A thousand beds were considered to be the maximum number an asylum should have, although many institutions, as in Leeds, Manchester and the South Western Metropolitan area, had twice this figure. The problem of overcrowding became much worse under the EMS war-time displacements and also when institutions were damaged by bombs. A detailed review in 1952 noted no new beds for mental patients in any areas, with serious defects in staff numbers and quality. The problem was exacerbated by an ageing population and, when RHB chairmen sought to expand their facilities, they commented that 'what we need is more money, more buildings, more steel and more staff – none of which seems likely to be available'. In his three years as

Minister of Health Iain Macleod acknowledged this to be his 'most difficult problem'; he gave it priority over everything else in the NHS and aimed to create an extra 2,800 beds in the service. However, it appears that spending on mental institutions in 1948–54 was £1m a year, less than half of the sum (£2.3m) that local authorities had expended in 1938–9. Recruiting campaigns for nursing staff failed, and by 1954 there were only 36 per cent registered mental nurses in the service, with the number of untrained staff doubling in the period 1949–56. Poor pay rates and working conditions resulted in an overtime ban early in 1956, the first nationwide industrial action under the NHS. By then, however, further health cuts were necessary as the defence budget expanded because of the Suez crisis.

The first new mental health facility to be built under the NHS was Greaves Hall, Liverpool, a mental deficiency institution for a thousand patients begun in 1953. Its first phase was completed five years later, to be followed by other developments at Balderton Hall, near Sheffield, Lea Castle, near Kidderminster and at Digby, near Exeter. The ageing population, however, was overtaking any such building programmes; the number of those over sixty-five in mental institutions was 16.4 per cent in 1944 but there were also a significant group (20 per cent) over seventy-five a decade later. To halt this trend, there was a move by the later 1950s towards increased outpatient services and community care for mental patients.

Primary care

From the earliest days when the Ministry of Health was formed in 1919 and the Dawson Report made its recommendations, there was a clear distinction between primary and secondary care. Primary care was seen as having both preventive and curative services linked into one organisation, to include the general practitioner, dental surgeon, pharmacist, nurse, midwife and health visitor. At the outset, the 20,000 GPs were the most forceful group within the NHS, for although they were well organised, especially on the matter of pay, they were individualists who resisted bureaucracy and conformity in their work. The collapse of the health centre movement in these early days was a mark of this individualism. GPs objected to capitation payments, which benefited practitioners with large lists who might, nevertheless, give a poorer service to so many patients. Practitioners who modernised their surgeries and facilities were not rewarded for such improvements.

In 1952 practitioners' salaries were raised to an average of £2,222 a year and the whole problem of lists was addressed. The theoretical maximum list was of 2,500 patients for a GP, but many practitioners had lists of 4,000, a breach that was widely condoned. Smaller lists would make it easier for new graduates to become established in practice and practitioners would be encouraged to move to understaffed areas of the country, although this was such a vexed question in the profession that the Medical Practices Committee was established to deal with it. The list maximum was finally agreed at 3,500, and some two million patients were reallocated to new practitioners to make this target figure possible. Smaller lists were allowed for rural areas. There were also plans to discourage single-handed and promote group practice, for the new arrangements were financially more advantageous to partners than to salaried assistants, many of whom were from overseas. The changes for GPs were noticeable. In 1952 there were 7,459 single-handed practitioners in England and Wales and 9,745 in partnerships; four years later these figures had changed to 6,691 and 12,272, an increase of 8 per cent in partnerships, a trend that continued into the next decade. The workloads that GPs carried varied considerably, although average statistics were gathered. However, in a large industrial town a single-handed practitioner could see between forty and fifty-five patients a day and make twenty-five house calls a day, as well as issuing some fifty sickness certificates in a week. Half a day off duty each week and other leisure time was usually negotiated with a neighbouring practice. A locum would be employed to cover an annual holiday fortnight.

There was also disquiet, in both the Treasury and the medical profession, about the proposal for an enforced retirement age of general practitioners to make openings for younger colleagues. In 1954 there were 1,188 GPs out of 18,513 (6.4 per cent) over the age of sixty-six and older practitioners wished to work on for ten years after 1948 to secure their superannuation benefits at retirement. More men and women were entering general practice as medical schools expanded and as hospital promotions were restricted, making many GPs anxious about competition and the government concerned at rising costs. It was felt that an extra seventy-five medical graduates a year would be needed to bring patient lists down to 2,000 and to cover the ageing British population. GPs themselves were also often in difficulties with their local hospitals, from which they were increasingly excluded and by whom they were regarded as 'glorified clerks'. As a move towards greater identity and to encourage education in general practice, the Royal College of General Practitioners was founded in 1952.

Health centres

The term 'health centre' was first used in the Dawson Report of 1920, with the idea of somewhere that would maintain health for the community rather than just cure illness. Health centres, of course, represented the very opposite of individuals in traditional practice. The idea became important to the Labour party from 1933. The term came to be used from 1939 for the new buildings that Local Health Authorities constructed and most practitioners disliked the concept because it inevitably involved receiving a salary from the LHA. However, health centres featured in section 21 of the 1946 NHS Act, which noted:

A main feature of the personal practitioner is to be the development of Health Centres. The object is that the Health Centre system should afford facilities for the general medical and dental services and also for many of the special clinic services of the local health authorities, and

sometimes also for out-post clinics of the hospitals and specialist services. The Centres will also serve as bases for various activities in health
education.

The BMA slowly accepted the idea and in a 1951 survey some 47 per cent of all
GPs acceded to the concept for the future.

However, the idea foundered. The most successful health centres were those
built for New Towns on green field sites, with six of the first seven built on new
housing estates where there were no established practices. The buildings were
usually cheaply constructed, with only the Woodberry Health Centre, Stoke
Newington, as a substantial showpiece costing £180,000. It was considered
extravagant and no more were built to this standard, although originally the
London County Council had planned 166 centres in their area. Harlow, with
four new centres, was the only community served by practitioners working exclusively from health centres. Those created in old communities, however, as at
Birmingham (Stechford) and Sheffield, collapsed in local rivalries. Bevan saw
the failure as a bitter humiliation, but in practical terms health centres neither
encouraged cooperation nor secured the GPs' support. The blame for their failure
was given to the Ministry of Health: medical politicians depicted them in a 'most
odious light', the Treasury was unwilling to find the substantial sums of money
required and building materials were desperately scarce. Even the well-known
establishment at Peckham was converted by the LCC into a recreation centre.

However, for all its difficulties, the NHS was essentially popular with the
British people and it became 'almost a part of the Constitution'. Undoubtedly
the medical profession feared loss of its independence and privileges, while the
whole question of charges was a watershed in both attitudes and administration.
On the tenth anniversary of the NHS, *The Times* commented that 'the nation
has good reason to be proud of the Health Service'. Whereas in 1939 there were
several different concepts and health schemes being considered, by the end of
the war, with unprecedented cooperation among various medical groups and
practical evidence that unification could work, a national scheme was virtually
inevitable. Although Labour was affronted by the concessions that were made to
the medical profession, particularly pay beds, merit awards, consultants' part
private practice and the continued autonomy of the teaching hospitals, the NHS
came into being as an ambitious publicly-funded compromise, rightly described
by Aneurin Bevan as 'the most civilised achievement of modern Government'.

Choose your doctor now

You and everyone in your family will be entitled to all usual advice and
treatment from a family doctor. Everyone aged 16 or over can choose his
or her own doctor. A family need not all have the same doctor, but parents
or guardians choose for children under 16.

Your dealings with your doctor will remain as they are now: *personal and confidential.* You will visit his surgery, or he will call on you, as may be necessary. The difference is that the doctor will be paid by the Government, out of funds provided by everybody.

Choose a doctor now – ask him to be your doctor under the new arrangements. Many will choose their present doctors. Any doctor can decline to accept a patient. If one doctor cannot accept you, ask another, or ask to be put in touch with one by the new "Executive Council" which has been set up in your area (you can get the address from the Post Office).

If you are already on a doctor's list under the old National Health Insurance Scheme, and if you do not wish to change your doctor, *do nothing.* Your name will stay on his list under the new Scheme.

But for your family, and for yourself if you are not already in the old National Health Insurance Scheme, now is the time to decide. Get an application form for *each* member of the family from the doctor you choose, or from any Post Office, Executive Council Office or public library. Fill in the forms and give them to the doctor.

Later your Executive Council will send a "medical card" to everyone who has been accepted by a doctor. If you want to change your doctor, you can do so at any time without difficulty. If you need a doctor when away from your own district, you can go to any doctor who is taking part in the new arrangements. You will not have to pay.

Help to have the Scheme ready by 5th July by choosing your doctor at once.

Ministry of Health leaflet, prepared in February 1948, for all households

Diary of a NHS baby: the 1950s

As a child I had a lot of ear infections and hated going to the doctor. Everything in the waiting room was brown. There was lino on the floor that was so highly polished that when you walked on it your shoes squeaked.

There was a deathly silence and you had to speak in whispers, but when you did everybody turned to look at you. There were no children's comics in the waiting room – it was always something like *Country Life.* I remember because I always used to look at the cottages that were for sale in the back. The seats were upright and made of brown leather and everything was in rows. For me as a child it was a forbidding place. I always hated going to the doctor after that. Even now, I'd much rather go to the dentist, although I have a super doctor and a modern surgery now ...

I remember queueing up for polio vaccinations at a hall in Lincoln where I grew up. We all stood in rows and I had the sugar cube, as you do now. It was a mass operation. I got a terrific thrill going to this because I watched *Emergency Ward 10* at the time and they had showed an iron lung with a person inside it. I had this terrific fear of polio, having seen what it could do to you. ... I remember the welfare orange juice they used to give me after cod liver oil. If you could get it now I would buy it. I think it was in a brown bottle but it was delicious. ... I remember Nitty Nora, the nurse who used to come round the schools to check for head lice. She was so rough, the way she used to pull your hair.

The Times, 23 June 1998

CONCLUSION

In the two centuries from 1750 to 1950 the advances in medicine can arguably be said to have had the greatest effect on most English lives, even more significant than universal education, both short and long term. Until the twentieth century limited medical skill and a lack of professional knowledge meant a high mortality rate in most illness, especially for the young, the pregnant and the old, while poor social conditions exacerbated sickness for most people for two hundred years. Medicine was essentially part of a consumer society until 1948, with the coming of state medicine in the National Health Service. In addition, the status of medical practitioners themselves and their profession has changed out of all recognition since 1750.

There is, however, a counter argument that medicine contributed little to any improvements in the country's health and that public disease-control methods were really responsible for lowered mortality and morbidity levels with the nineteenth century's control of the great epidemics. Such an argument, however, diminishes the importance of the many significant scientific discoveries of the period. New drugs, from digitalis, sulphonamides, arsenicals and penicillin to other new antibiotics, all indisputably saved lives. New medical equipment, including the clinical thermometer, the sphygmomanometer and X-rays, gave accurate diagnosis, alongside the development of laboratory and pathology services. New skills, especially in surgery, with improved anaesthesia, meant that more patients survived, while immunisation and vaccination came to prevent the major infections of children and adults. There were also clear improvements in psychiatric treatment and facilities across two centuries.

Although medical attention before the NHS was always linked to the ability to pay fees for treatment and afford drugs, it is now clear that a variety of systems existed in the eighteenth and nineteenth centuries that gave qualified medical attention to the mass of the population. Thus the many friendly societies provided medical care and sick pay to those above pauperism but never able to pay full professional fees, as well as access to their voluntary hospital, through institutional subscriptions, in many cases. The poor were also, as is clear from Overseers' accounts, attended by qualified men through the parish administration, again, in some instances, with access to the voluntary hospital and dispensary; they might even be seen by a physician in unusual circumstances. There were also by the nineteenth century a considerable range of dispensaries, free to the poorest, and piecemeal charity arrangements available, including vaccination and maternity facilities, as well as employers' and the hospitals' own schemes for poor patients. In 1911 the National Health Insurance scheme provided medical care for the largest homogeneous group of British citizens, lower wage-earners aged sixteen to seventy.

There has never been any suggestion, of course, that all these various groups of poorer patients received the same level of medical attention, although attended by the same practitioner, as the fee-paying, prosperous sufferers; some NHI panel patients recalled entering their GP's house by a separate side door. However, it was still possible for patients below the middle class to slip through the net and not to find medical attention through any of these means. The amalgamation of seventeen British provident associations to found BUPA in 1947, prior to the creation of the NHS, was to provide non-GP services for those who could not afford high private fees and did not belong to the NHI scheme. By 1950, when the NHS was fully functioning, BUPA had 50,000 registrations. The NHS, on the other hand, excluded no one, with medical attention free at the point of delivery, replacing what Charles Webster has called a 'ramshackle assemblage of health services' of the past.

While earlier ideas had been derided as utopian, the country's shared experiences of the Second World War had made possible a unified scheme and the destruction of many long-held, entrenched views, not least in the medical profession itself. During two centuries, patients' attitudes to practitioners changed beyond recognition. There had always been some sufferers with a cynically distrusting attitude – Byron remarked that 'the lancet had killed more people than the lance'. However, changes within medicine itself, bringing enhanced status and prosperity to practitioners, in turn gave consultants and GPs a place in society by the twentieth century that their predecessors could not have envisaged, except for the few grand physicians and 'surgeon princes' of earlier periods. The difficulties which have dogged the NHS in its first fifty years have virtually all rested on finance, with patients' rising expectations a crucial factor as both drugs and medical expertise reached levels unimagined in 1948. However, it is clear that health education has been relatively ineffective, so that, for example, Sir Richard Doll's findings on the links between smoking and lung cancer, published in 1952, have only slowly gained widespread acceptance after forty years. Modern medicine thus strives not only to cure but to prevent illness, perhaps the biggest change of all concepts in two centuries.

FURTHER READING

A number of titles are relevant to more than one topic and have accordingly been included in further reading for several chapters.
London is the place of publication unless otherwise stated.

Introduction: Medicine before the Industrial Revolution
Jonathan Andrews et al. (eds), The History of Bethlem, 1997.
W. F. Bynum and Roy Porter (eds), Companion Encyclopedia of the History of Medicine, 2 vols, 1997.
R. Campbell, The London Tradesman, 1747.
Charles Creighton, A History of Epidemics in Britain, 2 vols, 1965 edn.
Donald Hunter, Diseases of Occupations, 1974.
Joan Lane, John Hall and his Patients, Stroud, 1997.
A. Meiklejohn, 'John Darwall and "Diseases of Artisans"', British Journal of Industrial Medicine, 13, 1956.
Roy Porter, Heath for Sale, Manchester, 1989.
Roy Porter, The Greatest Benefit to Mankind, 1997.
Michael E. Rose, 'The doctor in the Industrial Revolution', Br. J. Industr. Med., 28, 1971.

Chapter 1: Medical practitioners in eighteenth- and nineteenth-century England
Brian Abel-Smith, The Hospitals, 1800–1948, 1964.
J. B. Bailey, The Diary of a Resurrectionist, 1896.
E. M. Brockbank, The Foundation of Provincial Medical Education in England, Manchester, 1936.
Bransby Blake Cooper, The Life of Sir Astley Cooper, 2 vols, 1843.
A. Cunningham and R. French (eds), The Medical Enlightenment of the Eighteenth Century, 1990.
Anne Digby, The Evolution of British General Practice, 1850–1948, Oxford, 1999.
Joan Lane, The Making of the English Patient: a guide to the sources for the social history of medicine, Stroud, 2000.
——, Apprenticeship in England, 1660–1914, 1997.
——, 'A provincial surgeon and his obstetric practice: Thomas W. Jones of Henley-in-Arden, 1764–1846', Medical History, 1987, 31, 3.
Irvine Loudon, Medical Care and the General Practitioner, 1750–1850, 1986.
Andrew Motion, Keats, 1997.
Vivian Nutton and Roy Porter, A History of Medical Education in Britain, Amsterdam, 1995.

Roy Porter and W. F. Bynum, *William Hunter and the Eighteenth-century Medical World*, 1983.
Ruth Richardson, *Death, Dissection and the Destitute*, 1987.
P. J. and R. V. Wallis, *Eighteenth-century Medics*, Newcastle upon Tyne, 1988.

Chapter 2: Population and contraception
David Davies, *The Case of Labourers in Husbandry*, 1795.
E. J. Dingwall, 'Early contraceptive sheaths', *British Medical Journal*, 3 January 1953.
David Gaimster *et al.*, 'The archaeology of private life: the Dudley Castle condoms', *Post-Medieval Archaeology*, **30**, 1996, 129–142.
Norman Himes, *A Medical History of Contraception*, New York, 1936.
Judith S. Lewis, *In the Family Way, 1760–1860*, New Brunswick, 1986.
R. W. Malcolmson, 'Infanticide in the eighteenth century' in J. S. Cockburn (ed.), *Crime in England, 1550–1800*, 1977.
T. McKeown, *The Modern Rise of Population*, 1976.
Angus McLaren, *A History of Contraception, from Antiquity to the Present Day*, 1990.
——, *Reproductive Rituals*, 1984.
——, *Birth Control in Nineteenth-century England*, 1978.
F. B. Smith, *The People's Health, 1830–1910*, 1979.

Chapter 3: Medical Care under the Old and the New Poor Law
P. Colquhoun, *A Treatise on Indigence*, 1806.
H. M. Colvin, *A Biographical Dictionary of British Architects, 1660–1840*, 1995.
Frank Crompton, *Workhouse Children: Infant and Child Paupers under the Worcestershire Poor Law, 1780–1871*, 1997.
Mary Anne Crowther, *The Workhouse System, 1834–1929*, 1981.
David Davies, *The Case of Labourers in Husbandry*, 1795.
Anna Dickens, 'The Architect and the Workhouse', *Architectural Review*, December 1976, 345–52.
Anne Digby, *Pauper Palaces*, 1978.
——, *Making a Medical Living*, Cambridge, 1994.
F. M. Eden, *The State of the Poor*, 3 vols, 1797.
Dorothy George, *London Life in the Eighteenth Century*, 1925.
Ruth G. Hodgkinson, *The Origins of the National Health Service: the Medical Services of the New Poor Law, 1834–1871*, 1967.
Dorothy Marshall, *The English Poor in the Eighteenth Century*, 1926.
Craig D. Stephenson, 'Victoria's Bastille? Solihull workhouse, 1836–1901', *Warwickshire History*, **VII**, 1, 1987.
Jeremy Taylor, *Hospital and Asylum Architecture in Britain, 1814–1914*, 1991.
Sidney and Beatrice Webb, *English Poor Law History*, parts 1 and 2, 1927, 1929.

Chapter 4: Medical care provided by Friendly Societies
J. Baernreither, *English Associations of Working Men*, 1889.
David Davies, *The Case of Labourers in Husbandry*, 1795.
F. M. Eden, *The State of the Poor*, 3 vols, 1797.
P. H. J. H. Gosden, *The Friendly Societies in England, 1815–1870*, Manchester, 1961.
D. Green, *Working Class Patients and the Medical Establishment*,1985.
R. P. Hastings, *Essays in North Riding history, 1780–1850*, Northallerton, 1981.

E. Posner, 'Eighteenth-century health and social service in the pottery industry of North Staffordshire', *Medical History*, 18, 2, April 1974.

James C. Riley, *Sick, not Dead*, 1977.

E. P. Thompson, *The Making of the English Working Class*, 1963.

See also the rules and records of many local friendly societies in county record offices.

Chapter 5: Hospitals and dispensaries

Gwendoline M. Ayers, *England's First State Hospitals and the Metropolitan Asylums Board, 1867–1930*, 1971.

Jonathan Barry and Colin Jones (eds), *Medicine and Charity Before the Welfare State*, 1991.

Fleetwood Buckle, *Vital and Economical Statistics of the Hospitals, Infirmaries etc of England and Wales for the year 1863*, 1863.

H. C. Burdett, *The Cottage Hospital, its Origin, Progress, Management and Work*, 1877.

Stephen Cherry, *Medical Services and the Hospital in Britain, 1860–1939*, 1996.

——, 'Before the National Health Service: financing the voluntary hospitals, 1900–39', *Econ. Hist. Review*, May 1997.

——, 'Beyond National Health insurance. The voluntary hospitals and hospital contributory schemes: a regional study, *Soc. Hist. of Medicine*, 5, 3, 1992.

Lindsay Granshaw and Roy Porter (eds), *The Hospital in History*, 1989.

F. K. Prochaska, *Philanthropy and the Hospitals of London: the King's Fund, 1897–1990*, Oxford, 1992.

Harriet Richardson (ed.), *English Hospitals, 1660–1948*, 1998.

M. Emrys Roberts, *The Cottage Hospitals, 1859–1990*, 1991.

Arnold Sorsby, 'Nineteenth-century provincial eye hospitals', *British Journal of Ophthalmology*, September 1946.

Jeremy Taylor, *The Architect and the Pavilion Hospital*, Leicester, 1997.

——, *Hospital and Asylum Architecture in England, 1840–1914*, 1991.

J. D. Thompson and G. Goldin, *The Hospital, a Social and Architectural History*, 1975.

John Woodward, *To do the Sick no Harm*, 1974.

Chapter 6: Asylums and prisons

Jonathan Andrews *et al.* (eds), *The History of Bethlem*, 1997.

E. M. Brockbank, 'Manchester's lead in the humane treatment of the insane', *B. M. J.*, 16 September 1933.

W. F. Bynum *et al.* (eds), *The Anatomy of Madness*, 2 vols, 1985.

Michael Clark and Catherine Crawford (eds), *Legal Medicine in History*, 1994.

H. M. Colvin, *Biographical Dictionary of British Architects, 1640–1840*, 1995.

John Duncumb, *Collections Towards the History and Antiquities of Herefordshire*, 2 vols, 1804–12.

Anne Digby, *Madness, Morality and Medicine: a Study of the York Retreat, 1796–1914*, Cambridge, 1985.

Thomas R. Forbes, *Surgeons at the Bailey*, Yale, 1985.

Francis and Charles Fox, *History and Present State of Brislington House*, Bristol, 1836.

Charles G. M. Gaskell, *Passages in the History of York Lunatic Asylum, 1772–1901*, Wakefield, 1902.

Elizabeth Hamilton, *The Warwickshire Scandal*, Norwich, 1999.

R. P. Hastings, *Essays in North Riding History, 1780–1850*, 1981.

John Howard, *The State of the Prisons in England and Wales*, Warrington, 1780.

Richard Hunter and Ida Macalpine, *Psychiatry for the Poor*, 1974.

——, *Three Hundred Years of Psychiatry, 1535–1860*, New York, 1982.

Richard Hunter et al., 'The County Register of houses for the reception of "Lunatics", 1798–1812', *Jnl of mental sciences*, 1956.

Michael Ignatieff, *A Just Measure of Pain*, 1978.

Alan Ingram (ed.), *Patterns of Madness in the Eighteenth Century*, Liverpool, 1998.

A. W. Langford, 'The history of Hereford General Hospital', *Woolhope Naturalists' Field Club Transactions*, **XXXVI**, 1958–60.

Anthony Masters, *Bedlam*, 1977.

W. Ll. Parry-Jones, *The Trade in Lunacy*, 1972.

Nikolaus Pevsner, appropriate county volumes of *The Buildings of England*.

Roy Porter, *Mind Forg'd Manacles*, 1987.

Harriet Richardson (ed.), *English Hospitals, 1660–1948*, 1998.

Andrew T. Scull, *Museums of Madness*, 1979.

L. D. Smith, 'The pauper lunatic problem in the West Midlands, 1815–1850, *Midland History*, **XXI**, 1996.

——, *'Cure, Comfort and Safe Custody': Public Lunatic Asylums in Nineteenth-century England*, Leicester, 1999.

Jeremy Taylor, *Hospital and Asylum Architecture in England, 1840–1914*, 1991.

Samuel Tuke, *Description of The Retreat, an Institution near York for Insane Persons of the Society of Friends*, York, 1813.

David Wright, 'Getting out of the asylum: understanding the confinement of the insane in the nineteenth century', *Soc. Hist. of Medicine*, **10**, 1, April 1997.

The Medical Times and Gazette, **1**, 5 March 1870.

Select Committee on the State of Lunatics (Criminal and Pauper), 1807 (39), **II**.

Chapter 7: Midwifery and nursing

Brian Abel-Smith, *A History of the Nursing Profession*, 1960.

James H. Aveling, *English Midwives, their History and Prospects*, 1872.

Celia Davies (ed.), *Rewriting Nursing History*, 1980.

Robert Dingwall, Anne Marie Rafferty and Charles Webster, *An Introduction to the Social History of Nursing*, 1988.

Jean Donnison, *Midwives and Medical Men*, New York, 1977.

Christopher J. Maggs, *The Origins of General Nursing, 1881–1914*, 1983.

Christopher J. Maggs (ed.), *Nursing History: the State of the Art*, 1987.

Hilary Marland, *The Art of Midwifery*, 1993.

Judith Moore, *A Zeal for Responsibility: the Struggle for Professional Nursing in Victorian England, 1868–83*, 1988.

Hugh Small, *Florence Nightingale, Avenging Angel*, 1998.

Anne Marie Rafferty, *The Politics of Nursing Knowledge*, 1996.

Jean Towler and Joan Bramall, *Midwives in History and Society*, 1986.

Percival Willoughby, *Observations in Midwifery*, 1863 edn.

Adrian Wilson, *The Making of Man-midwifery*, 1995.

Chapter 8: Infections and disease control

Paul-Gabriel Boucé (ed.), *Sexuality in Eighteenth-century Britain*, Manchester, 1982.

Charles Creighton, *A History of Epidemics in Britain*, 2 vols, 1965 edn.

S. L. Cummins, *Tuberculosis in History*, 1949.

Thomas Dormandy, *The White Death: a History of Tuberculosis*, 1999.

Michael Durey, *The Return of the Plague: Cholera, 1831–2*, Dublin, 1979.

David Evans, 'Tackling the "Hideous Scourge": the creation of the VD treatment centres in early 20th century Britain', *Social History of Medicine*, **5**, 3, December 1992.

Anne Hardy, *The Epidemic Streets: Infectious Disease and the Rise of Preventive Medicine, 1856–1900*, Oxford, 1993.

Alethea Hayter, 'The sanitary idea and a Victorian novelist', *History Today*, December 1969.

G. Melvyn Howe, *People, Environment, Disease and Death*, Cardiff, 1997.

Joan Lane, ' "A little purging and bleeding": poverty and disease in eighteenth-century Stratford', in Robert Bearman (ed.), *The history of an English borough*, Stroud, 1997.

McKeown, Thomas, *The Modern Rise of Population*, 1976.

Linda E. Merians (ed.), *The Secret Malady*, Kentucky, 1996.

R. J. Morris, *Cholera, 1832*, 1976.

Ronald Paulson, *Hogarth*, **1**, **2**, New Brunswick, 1991.

Peter Razzell, *The Conquest of Smallpox*, Firle, 1977.

S. M. Tomkins, 'Venereal prophylaxis debate in Britain, 1916–26', *Medical History*, **37**, 4, October 1993.

Bridget A. Towers, 'Health education policy, 1916–26', *Medical History*, **24**, 1, January 1980.

A. S. Wohl, *Endangered Lives: Public Health in Victorian Britain*, 1984.

Chaper 9: The pharmaceutical industry

Juanita G. L. Burnby, *A Study of the English Apothecary from 1660 to 1760*, Medical History Supplement, no. 3, 1983.

William Chamberlaine, *Tyrocinium Medicum: or a Dissertation on the Duties of Youth Apprenticed to the Medical Profession*, 1819.

Stanley Chapman, *Jesse Boot of Boots the Chemists*, 1973.

Desmond Chapman-Huston, *Through a City Archway, the Story of Allen and Hanbury, 1715–1954*, 1954.

Robert Rhodes James, *Henry Wellcome*, 1994.

Gilbert Macdonald, *One Hundred Years: Wellcome, 1880–1980*, 1980.

G. Macfarlane, *Alexander Fleming, the Man and the Myth*, 1984.

Leslie G. Matthews, *History of Pharmacy in Britain*, Edinburgh, 1962.

Thomas Richards, *The Commodity Culture of Victorian England: Advertising and Spectacle, 1851–1914*, Stanford, 1991.

Geoffrey Tweedale, *At the Sign of the Plough*, 1990.

J. R. Vane, 'The research heritage of Henry Wellcome', *Pharmaceutical Historian*, **10**, 2, August 1980.

See also the pharmaceutical data base at the Wellcome Institute Library, London and local trade directories for the nineteenth century.

Chapter 10: Medicine and war

Tony Ashworth, *Trench Warfare, 1914–1918, the Live and Let Live System*, 1980.

Anthony Babington, *For the Sake of Example*, 1985.

John Blair, *Centenary History of the Royal Army Medical Corps*, 1998.

Gay Braybon and Penny Summerfield, *Out of the Cage: Women's Experiences in Two World Wars*, 1987.

Vera Brittain, *Testament of Youth*, 1933.

Neil Cantlie, *A History of the Army Medical Department*, 2 vols, 1974.

Roger Cooter, Mark Harrison and Steve Sturdy (eds), *Medicine and Modern Warfare*, Amsterdam, 1999.

Roger Cooter, *Surgery and Society in Peace and War*, Manchester, 1993.

E. J. Dennison, *A Cottage Hospital Grows Up*, 1993.

L. F. Haber, *The Poisonous Cloud: Chemical Warfare in the First World War*, 1986.

C. B. Heald, *Genesis of Aviation Medicine in the Fighting Services of the Royal Flying Corps and the Royal Air Force*, typescript, RAF Museum, Hendon, 0277 94.

Leah Leneman, 'Medical women at war, 1914–18', *Medical History*, **38**, 2, Apr 1994.

Lyn Macdonald, *The Roses of No Man's Land*, 1980.

Harriet Richardson (ed.), *English Hospitals, 1660–1948*, 1998.

J. M. Winter, 'The impact of World War I on civilian health in Britain', *Economic History Review*, **XXX,** no. 3, August 1977.

——, 'Military fitness and civilian health in Britain during the First World War', *Journal of Contemporary History*, **XV,** 2.

Jay Winter, *The Great War and the British People*, 1995.

Jeremy Taylor, *Hospital and Asylum Architecture in England, 1840–1914*, 1991.

Regiment, special issue of the magazine for the RAMC centenary, May 1998.

Chapter 11: The National Health Service

Brian Abel-Smith, *The NHS: the First Thirty Years*, 1978.

P. W. J. Bartrip, *Mirror of Medicine: a History of the BMJ*, Oxford, 1990.

Virginia Berridge, *Health Policy and Health, 1939–1997*, 1998.

J. Carrier and I. Kendall, *Health and the NHS*, 1998.

Anne Digby and Nick Bosanquet, 'Doctors and patients in an era of national health insurance and private practice, 1913–38', *Economic History Review*, XLI, no.1, February 1988.

Derek Fraser, *The Evolution of the British Welfare State*, 1973.

David Gladstone (ed.), *Before Beveridge: Welfare Before the Welfare State*, 1999.

George Godber, *The NHS, Past, Present and Future*, 1975.

Andrew Land et al., *The Development of the Welfare State, 1939–1951*, HMSO, 1992 .

Jane Lewis, *What Price Community Medicine?*, 1986.

R. Lowe, *The Welfare State in Britain Since 1945*, 1993.

F. N. L. Poynter, *The Evolution of Medical Practice in Britain*, 1961.

John Stewart, 'Socialist proposals for health reform in inter-war Britain: the case of Somerville Hastings', *Medical History*, 39, 3, July 1995.

Pat Thane, *Foundations of the Welfare State*, 1996.

Charles Webster, *The National Health Service, a political history*, 1998.

——, *The Health Services since the War*, vol. 1, *Problems of Health Care: the National Health Service Before 1957*, 1988.

INDEX OF PLACES

INDEX OF MEDICAL NAMES

a. = after   b. = before   d. = died   n.d. = no dates known

SUBJECT INDEX

Printed in the United States
by Baker & Taylor Publisher Services

Printed in the United States
by Baker & Taylor Publisher Services